Before the Curtain Opens

Before the Curtain Opens

Alexander Technique
in the Actor's Life

Kate Kelly

Published in this first edition in 2018 by:
Triarchy Press
Axminster, England

info@triarchypress.net
www.triarchypress.net

A catalogue record for this book is available from the British Library

ISBN: 978-1-911193-43-2

Printed and bound in Great Britain by
TJ International Ltd, Padstow, Cornwall

For Daniel
and
for my family

"Everything has been written before, but not by me"
Giles Vigneault

Acknowledgements

Thank you to the great group of artists from three different countries who so very kindly stepped up and gave of their talents to illustrate this book: Jim Cahill, Luc Chamberland, Michael Hegarty, Vivien Kelly, Dee Shulman, Lucinda Sieger, Marie Eve Tanguay.

I would like to give particular thanks to my two life teachers Walter Carrington and Hilmar Schonauer, from whom I have learned so much.

Thank you to my secondary school English teacher Miss Brigid Murray.

To those who gave me very practical initial feedback and advice on the text, thank you: Monique Vanormelingen for first addressing my idiosyncratic grammar and spelling; FEU Equity writers workshop; Jerry Sontag; and Steven Hallmark.

Thank you also to Moya Henry, Nica Gimeno, Marie Claude Maisoneuve Quellen for past collaborations; to Jean Fischer and Regina Stratil, who pinpointed some elusive research; to Marjorie Hodge and Chantal Marsolais, who both told me to get on with it.

Thank you to the first readers who also encouraged me: Mary Holland, Barbara Darnley, Sandra Leal, Julie Barber, Andreas Sandri and especially my husband Daniel Tanguay without whom this book would never have been written.

Like the best of theatre directors, my editor, Andrew, has guided this first-time author with kindness, skill and sensitivity, with just enough nudges to keep me improving, for which I am very grateful.

Illustrations

Cover image: Luc Chamberland

'Bath', p. 4: Dee Shulman

'Star', p. 17: Luc Chamberland

'Heel bone', p. 31: Marie Eve Tanguay

'Misericord', p. 38: Michael Hegarty

'Tight rope walker', p. 46: Luc Chamberland

'Lying down position', p. 55: Jim Cahill

'Tree', p. 64: Vivien Kelly

'Chair', p. 82: Lucinda Sieger

Drawing of F. M. Alexander, p.87: Joanne Emma. Copyright Jean M. O. Fischer © 2015

Image of the author, p. 113: Daniel Tanguay

Contents

Preamble

I cannot remember when I first wanted to become an actor but I do know the moment when I realised the Alexander technique had cheerfully and thoroughly inveigled its way into my life.

As a young actor, I had lessons in the technique which bolstered my confidence and gave me a greater sense of myself. They were also so enjoyable that I think I took all the subtle changes quite for granted.

A few years later, passing on my experience in European theatre, I was giving a very physically based workshop to actors in Belfast when suddenly I wanted them all to stop doing things and just lie down. Oh no, I thought, I want to teach them the Alexander technique… a bolt from the blue like a vocational calling. I was quite cross as I had thought I was happy enough as an actor. Some months later, however, I moved to London to begin my training as an Alexander teacher.

In a sequel, all these years later, I recently found myself working with another group of young actors, who gradually discovered, after a series of Alexander lessons, a new awareness of unnoticed habits and available choices in their daily lives.

I told them how cavalry cadets on receiving the command to canter can learn to collect themselves momentarily while thinking "I have time" before they pass on the order, ensuring a smooth and free movement transition for their horse.[1]

The actors riding their own horse, as it were, discovered that something as simple as learning how to stop the

---

[1] As told in Walter Carrington (1994) *Thinking Aloud.*

unconscious habit of tensing their neck muscles in reaction to a thought or a situation, at intervals during the day, improved the fluidity and coordination of even small movements.

Remembering at the same time the upward flow of the energy in the body is not only relaxing but allows them to speedily change their mind about moving or reacting, without startling 'their horse'.

Because of this repeated experience, they can find, in years to come, creative choices influenced and enriched in all areas of their professional stage and screen work. The opportunity is there to support performance without the interference of unnecessary stress.

For those not in training or well past that level it can sometimes be difficult to know how you can renew the energising and calming effects of a lesson, or even why it is important to take lessons in the first place... This book will remind you.

I invite you to read it to accompany your understanding and application of the technique in your life. Although it is primarily written for actors, its message is helpful to all types of performers and any current or potential student (or 'pupil' as you are called by your teacher) of the Alexander technique.

It may be that you will not take Alexander lessons nor ever stand on a stage but for the general reader this book also offers useful references and guidance for everyday situations.

After all, if life is not a rehearsal then it is the performance, and so we are all performers in the act of living.

P.S. Frederic Matthias Alexander (more of him later) of the technique's name is referred to in this book simply as F.M. as he was known in his social circle.

Before

Long before the curtain opens on your performance, the creative impulse is nestling in the everyday awaiting its opportunity to surprise you.

However, at the same time as going about your daily life you are unwittingly under the sway of the very habits and attitudes that will compromise your individual creative expression.

This book addresses the conundrum and how you can be conscious, alert and ready – "The readiness is all" being one of F.M. Alexander's favourite Shakespeare quotes – so that, when inspiration strikes, you can carry it through, without impediment, into your characterisation and performance.

If morning rituals involve unnoticed muscle tightening and breath holding, a small snowball of unnecessary tensions starts to roll down the snowy slope of the day faster and faster arriving at the bottom of the hill (performance time) as a much larger snowball. You can easily find yourself having to deal with all that accumulated stress at the same time as you are coping with any nervousness about stepping into the spotlight.

True to its title this book is all about 'Before'. Everything that happens before the curtain rises. Before you bend over to tie up your shoe laces, before you read out loud, even before that impulse which mysteriously propels you to arrive at the characterisation for your acting role. 'Before' doesn't remain neatly in a tidy past; it is a potent force which spills over into the present and future.

It is also the springboard for your creative trajectory, your starting point: how you are in the everyday, your attitudes, how you respond to all that is around and within you.

Without the 'springiness', inspiration falls flat fast, the bubbles can't fizz. There isn't anything to sustain any momentary imaginative leap.

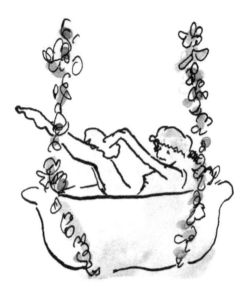

The more you learn to pay attention to your experiences, decision-making and approach to life, the greater depth and potential you lend to your talent and skills as a performer. This may be what makes the difference between the flash-in-the-pan creative and having an enduring and renewing quality of artistry.

Happily, 'Before' features quite strongly in the teaching of the Alexander technique, enabling your foundation or starting point to be sturdy so your constructs have integrity and can be sustained without strain. This establishes a reliable underpinning for your vision and inspiration.

As with preparing to play a violin, with the Alexander technique you learn to fine-tune your own instrument (yourself) checking on nuances in your thought patterns and responses and their influence on the choices you make. In a very practical way you discover how to use your intention to affect physicality, breathing, emotions, voice and attitude and to prevent unhelpful, unnoticed habits of tension from stymying your expression.

As a young actor, I had the opportunity to work with an international theatre research company in Europe. Members of the company were given a lot of responsibility to create and devise. The way we worked with our director was, I believe, similar to the way her dancers worked with Pina Bausch: suggesting projects/enacted ideas that could be developed for a themed production. I created striking, extravagant images including descending from the Flies in a full-sized bath tub to illustrate a scene in Dante's Divine Comedy. It is not surprising to me that I failed in my attempts to incorporate text into my creation. I hadn't connected with what was needed to sustain my expression beyond the excitement of manifesting my imagination in this way. Looking back on it, I had little awareness of how the 'Before' of my everyday life was impacting on my creative choices. I didn't have sufficient breadth of experience or understanding to go beyond the initial 'flash'.

Whether or not you are responsible for creating your own scripts or scenes, experience shows that the only person you the actor can rely upon is yourself. Not the director, nor fellow players. Sometimes not even the playwright or script writer and certainly not the harassed assistant stage manager who sets out your props on stage... or doesn't. If you can learn to inhabit the full stature of yourself in all areas of your life, you will have an infinite source of capability to rely upon.

'Before' encompasses everything that goes on in life, noticed and unnoticed. The following chapters are a resource of notes and reflections to draw on as you build your personal foundation of self-reliance and awareness to ensure the bubbles keep bubbling in life and performance.

Habit

When nervous, overtired, under stress or ill, everyone has the tendency to display an exaggerated version of their patterns of habit. This is something you have in common with your audience who, for the most part, if asked to walk across a stage in front of a hall full of people (as, for instance, at a graduation ceremony) would probably feel and look quite awkward and, in an effort to appear 'natural', quite stiff. The idiosyncrasies inherent in movement become very obvious.

What may separate the amateur from the professional, however, is the need for extensive self-appraisal and a recognition of how much work is required to match the wish with the reality. One of Alexander's aphorisms was "You think you are doing what you think you are doing but you are not". In other words, I have the idea to take a step in a certain style and I think I have done so, but in fact I have put into action my habitual manner of moving, superimposed the new idea and gained only a superficial change.

The sort of actor content with this 'acting-lite' approach has been referred to quite aptly by the late Bertie Scott as a 'Strummer' or as a 'Personality Actor', "one that thinks their personality will satisfy all demands". [2]. In other words, someone who enacts on stage only what he does during the day, limiting himself to habitual unnoticed patterns of reaction and action. Several of these may be endearing, recognisable and large enough to sustain a characterisation that can be, to a certain extent, successful. But it becomes one

---

[2] Bertie Scott (1964) *The Life of Acting*, Bertie Scott Memorial Foundation.

that is repeated with little variety whatever role is played.

This is completely different from familiar individual *qualities* 'showing through'. The audience may identify them with the actor, yet these qualities enhance a role and carry the expression of the actor's intent beyond the habitual. They are present at all times and are a mark of the inner life of a person. This may also be what makes some of the greatest performances so memorable.

Unnoticed or unconscious habits pervade our daily lives and thank goodness for many of them... we don't have to think through every movement we make. The muscles have blueprints stored away for a myriad possible actions. Yet, if creativity is dependent on free choice, unhelpful habits begin to interfere with the process and it is not too fanciful to say that they make the choices for us.

What is it about habit that gets in our way? First and foremost, it is an attitude, often a fixed way of seeing ourselves and the world around us. This translates into limited imaginative choices and even stiffness in movement.

Unnoticed habit becomes the dead end for creativity. It hampers the connection between imagination and expression. The only way this cul-de-sac can be avoided is if habit is identified and a stop put to these patterns of thought and activity.

In order to change this you must learn how to stop the habit. Anyone who has ever experimented with changing a routine as simple as how to brush your teeth or your hair will know it's not quite as easy as it sounds. (More, however, will follow on how the Alexander technique can make it possible).

It is already clear that however you are during the day can, if not checked, inform if not dictate how you reveal yourself in character in performance. Louis Malle's 1981 film 'My Dinner with Andre' encapsulates much of what I believe about theatre and life. It takes place over a meal involving not an intellectual discussion but a dialogue of storytelling between the two protagonists, played by Wallace Shawn and

Andre Gregory. They journey through uncertainty, scepticism, doubt and humanity from two very different starting points. The characters agree on what is needed and not needed in both life and art. "When people just concentrate on their goals in life, life becomes habitual, they live each moment by habit. If you're operating by habit you're not really living."

Which leads me again to the conclusion that operating by habit in life (where you are not living fully) will inevitably translate into a performance and a characterisation not fully inhabited. You cannot expect to make the leap from a habitually lived life to a habit-free performance in the time it takes to walk from your dressing room to the performance space.

It is everything that happens 'Before' in your off-stage life that transforms how and what you achieve in performance.

Life? or Theatre?

A very powerful example of the interdependence and inter-linkedness of life and art, the force of art motivating life and life becoming art, is displayed in the permanent exhibition of paintings at the Jewish Historical Museum in Amsterdam called 'Life? or Theatre?' by Charlotte Salomon. She undertook this massive and rich artwork (the total collection is 800 gouaches) recounting the story of her Berlin Jewish family, in little under a year before her untimely death in 1943 and painted scenes from her life, with overlays of words and melodies, created a poster introducing the characters, added a narrator, invited an imaginary audience, and announced the setting of the play. Her life made operatic. Inspired by her stepmother's extraordinary singing teacher Alfred Wolfsohn, the energy and impact behind her art motivated her life choices. The two became indivisible.

This same source of exultation in life and art ultimately produced the pioneering Roy Hart theatre[3] whose members in working with the 8 Octave voice demand the same commitment to everyday living as to performance. The energy of theatre strongly echoed in life. This is about living fully. By challenging the voice to attain extremes of (literally) highs and lows a Roy Hart actor (or workshop student) not only extends the range of their voice beyond the small band of sound used for 'normal' or habitual speech but the sounds emitted by self and others in a group singing lesson simultaneously awaken the heart and energise the will and imagination.

---

[3] https://roy-hart-theatre.com

The habitual has no part to play in these experiences and yet I found it was still there in me, despite it being pushed quite strongly to the sidelines, because it had not been fully consciously addressed. It was, however, the discovery of my voice's potential, as a younger actor, particularly the lessons I received from Marita Gunther, Jonathan Hart and especially Ivan Midderigh of the Roy Hart Theatre that propelled me towards a fuller life and eventually the training to become an Alexander teacher.

So how is it that the Alexander technique can change what even this tremendous artistic force could not shift or sustain in me?

I think it may be because you learn nothing new with the Alexander technique. Instead it awakens inherent knowledge in the senses and sinews of the self. It is getting right back to original basics, to the foundation that will support everything else: your voice, your expression, your vivacity.

In your Alexander lessons you are taught a practical method to remember what you have forgotten and what you innately knew as a small child. Memory is in every cell in the body. The musculature can let out a sigh. "Ah yes I remember this, it's easier this way." That's why your first encounter with the technique during a hands-on lesson can sometimes be a very relaxing experience and give you an 'Aha' moment.

Walking down the road after my first Alexander appointment with Glynn MacDonald I was floating on air feeling both utterly transformed and more myself – a most addictive feeling. Perhaps this is one of the reasons why David Boxer, an acting tutor when I was a drama school student, had told us all that "the Alexander technique is like gold dust".

The challenge may come a little later, after your first few lessons. Then you have to choose between what has become, over the years, comfortable and expected and the conscious application of the principles of the technique that connect you with what is simply natural but not 'the usual'. At first, learning to overcome the old habitual reactions that interfere with this process isn't necessarily an easy attitude to maintain.

What F.M. discovered was that in order to restore this connection and, in this instance, change the way he was talking on stage (which was causing hoarseness) he had to begin by stopping whatever it was he was doing, i.e. speaking. He didn't try to superimpose a new vocal technique onto the old way. He simply stopped the habitual pattern by refusing to cooperate with the impulse. The muscles all ready to organise themselves for utterance mode 'stood down'.

He then subtly brought about the reorganisation of the musculature in his neck, head and back and made a choice to speak or not speak.

This intervention of stopping he called 'Inhibition' but please do not mistake Inhibition for 'suppression'. The energy of the impulse still remains and is not repressed. There is simply time created for a choice to be made as to how that energy is to be used – in this example of whether to speak or not to speak.[4]

I have found that if I take an 'educated moment' to inhibit any usual preparation before reading out loud (the clearing of the throat, posing the head, taking a deep breath, etc.) and approach it instead with some Alexander instruction, the clarity and sound of my voice is changed for the better.

In the split second before you make the conscious decision to perform an action your musculature has already prepared itself for the activity without you consciously choosing how to do so. This handy blueprint has, however, turned out to have developed a slight flaw, involving over-tension of muscle, that needs amendment. That's why merely deciding

[4] For a good explanation of the difference between suppression and Inhibition, see Frank Pierce Jones (1997) *Freedom to Change*, Mouritz, p.14.

to perform the action differently from usual won't work, as the muscles then receive conflicting messages.

F.M.'s genius was in discovering empirically what was proven over 70 years later in the laboratory[5] and it is our luck that he showed us the practical means to overcome the power of unconscious habit.

His discovery quickly changed the nature of his own performances. His breathing became less audible and his voice was consistently clear and strong. Other actors and singers came for help to improve their own vocal capacities and so began the development of what became the technique that is taught today.

In your Alexander lessons you recover what F.M. went on to find: that the natural upward release against the gravitational pull is ensured when your neck muscles are free (not tight) and the head balances on top of the spine (not held or retracted). The head leads the way so that the body follows it upwards while the back and torso are expanded and at a natural length. F.M. called this relationship between the neck, head and back the 'Primary Control'. When its interrelated balance is interfered with, little else can work efficiently.

It is only after you have taken time to consciously re-establish this finely tuned interrelationship and made a choice to speak (or perform any other action) that your muscles can proceed to engage from this new starting point. In this process there is no extra 'doing' activity, only directed thought.

Although this sounds like a long, tedious procedure to learn and put into action, it is not. It follows a forgotten natural rhythm and pathway that eventually feels 'normal' again.

---

[5] Benjamin Libet's 1965 experiments in the timing of consciousness. For more information, see www.consciousentities.com/libet.htm

F.M.'s discoveries depend on the fact that all nerve pathways leaving the brain directly or indirectly affect muscle. Everything you think will influence your muscle. Even while reading a book, muscles are enlivened as imagination takes you into the descriptive action or dialogue. (Reading or watching a screen for a length of time, however, can over-stimulate the nervous system and musculature, leading to a loss of focus).[6]

With the Alexander technique you are harnessing the energy of thought in a very specific way. This he called 'Direction'. You direct the thought for the neck to be free, for the head to go forward and up, the back to lengthen and widen. (Not to be confused with stage directions often found in *italics* in a script.)

It is necessary to be precise in the wording of these instructions/directions (or polite requests) for the brain to become accustomed to accepting and acting upon them. Energy will then follow the thought. For actors who understand how much the power of 'Intention' influences their acting this is not such a difficult concept to grasp.

Just as for F.M., for me and hundreds of thousands of others, you will find that, as you practise Inhibition and Direction, any muscular holding will gradually respond to directed thought more easily and habit's hold will be loosened, in both theatre and life.

There is no 'one fits all' right way to do anything, but plenty of wrong ways. This is what the Alexander technique teaches you to prevent. To stop the wrong thing (the interfering habit) so the right thing can 'do itself' or as the late Robin Williams put it, "What's right is what's left if you do everything else wrong."

---

6 https://www.theguardian.com/books/2014/dec/23/ebooks-affect-sleep-alertness-harvard-study

Starbursts of Stopping

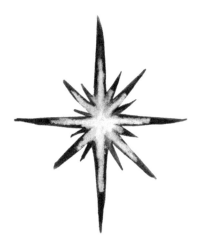

Stopping/Inhibition is not stopping dead or freezing on the spot; nor is it a long process. We are talking seconds and split seconds each time. It is a moment of poise and expansion where there is a deliberate suspension of activity before a decision 'to do or not to do' is made. For a hummingbird to remain in one place in the air while it drinks nectar from a flower, its wings 'flap' an average 50 times per second. Our energetic system is just as enlivened in this moment of stillness, as in action. It is a starburst of space that gives a possibility, a creative opportunity. Every time you decide not to do an action in the usual way and then use directed thought, you reinforce and explore a new approach rather than falling into the trench of old habit.

Energy

During her Alexander lessons, Lucinda, a singer, composer and artist, experienced lightness and the sense of going up towards the stratosphere. Without gravity, however, this direction of going upwards would leave her ungrounded, unearthed. Gravity provides the stabiliser, the balancing force that keeps her feet on the ground as she continues to 'rise'.

While Lucinda has the ability to balance and not fall over, she can literally go up in the opposite direction from gravity during walking, drawing or singing. In other words, while living her life. This is her – and every healthy human's – birth right. Anti-gravity responses activated in muscle/spine/brain pathways are designed, when we are in the upright, to propel us upwards.

These and the life energy within us counter what could become the overwhelming effects of gravity, especially when we are over-tired or unthinking.

A variety of factors in early childhood – imitating adults, sitting on furniture not designed for humans (let alone children), as well as being startled – begin to compromise and interfere with this innate ability.

Apprehension eventually appears to become physically manifested, even when it is not called for and develops into a mental and physical attitude that dictates how to move in the simplest of activities like sitting, standing, walking, talking and even breathing.

The root of this is, not surprisingly, often referred to as 'Startle Pattern', easily identifiable when a random selection of pedestrians walk past a building site and the shock of a sudden very loud noise causes them all (to a greater or lesser extent) to retract the head, stiffen neck muscles, raise shoulders and momentarily hold their collective breath. No one chooses to react in this way, it is visceral and feels automatic – left over from a time when fight or flight were the only options. While it may physiologically prepare us for action if needed, many of us instead become stuck in 'fright'. Without realising it, after the shock has passed, a diluted version of the physical reminder of it can remain for some time, reinforcing the pattern we are already unconsciously living by.

What could prevent Lucinda from performing at her most creative is this embedded experience of retraction replayed over and over in the day. It might also stop her sketching from evolving new qualities. In this 'pulling down with gravity' mode, she would regularly draw a line downwards towards the bottom of the page, which can cause a loss of the artist's hand coordination and control, whereas going up with the line makes the process easier and freer and encourages the flow of inspiration to be unimpeded.

With an economic use of energy, multi-tasking as a performer can be very nurturing of your talents: the actor who writes stories, the performer who directs, the singer and artist like Lucinda who not only composes her own music but has an ongoing creative life at her finger tips.

One creative activity feeds another. Time for less busyness is, however, essential. A regrouping of energy from time to time is vital. Some performers also really need the space and time to bake cakes, oil an engine, plant a garden. This time away from the 'day job' allows the unconscious to process information and 'back stories' already absorbed or studied. Realisations and understanding pop up while the conscious mind is otherwise seemingly occupied. It may seem surprising that clear creative choices are often shaped from this place. Lin-Manuel Miranda, the creator of the musical 'Hamilton', reminds himself that "the good idea comes when you are walking your dog, or in the shower or waking up from sleep."[7]

The fabulous informed unconscious will have its own 'on-stage' moment during the 'spaces in between' (see page 73).

Rather thrillingly, John Upledger posits that certain molecules (protein) in the body have intellect and are busily supporting your creative self like so many in-house artistic consultants:

> They simply make hundreds of thousands of judgment calls every minute that you are alive. ... I also strongly suspect they have feelings, *creative tendencies* and that they probably respond to an environment that is conscious in a very positive and optimistic way.[8]

Paul Scofield, one of the finest actors of the 20th century, understood the parameters of his own energy very well. He wrote:

> Output in the theatre requires greater energy than anything else I know. Doubt of one's energy is the worst of all. One's output in the theatre requires energy of a sort that is never a factor in family life. Family energy generates itself. Social life outside the family can be exhausting.[9]

Tiredness, or when you haven't taken enough time to stop, easily pulls you down into the habitual pattern of a 'reduced' startle pattern. No one looks after the actor and their energy except the actor himself. Recognise the space and time you need as an individual to 'be at your best'.

Find your own balance between activities and rest. Acknowledge the people, situations and recreational pursuits that sap your vitality and get in the way of your

---

[7] *Observer* Newspaper interview, 10 December 2017.

[8] John Upledger, (2003) *Cell Talk*, North Atlantic Books.

[9] H.K. Chinoy and T. Cole (1970) *Actors on Acting*, Three Rivers.

work. My friend Wilfrid Murray, concert pianist and Alexander teacher, told me that, in order to focus on a serious two-hour piano practice session, he needs a further two hours either side with little of import happening. I was immensely relieved to hear this as I at last understood my need to 'faff around' before I could settle to my writing and indeed, in the past, line learning. It's not always about overcoming a resistance but about attuning to the creative matter in hand.

You may be one of the lucky 'ready tuned' performers who can seem to switch from the social interchange to creative engagement in a turn of the head. It may be however that you 'think yourself' into the space you need, in advance. You have found a happy balance.

If this is not your way then explore a change in rhythm, take more time for yourself and note what kind of energy usually keeps you going and if it expands or contracts your creative possibilities. Do not mistake nervous energy – adrenaline sourced – for your vital life energy.

That buzzy feeling can do a temporary job in urgent circumstances but, like a 'sugar high', it does not sustain you, with discernment, for long. Perpetual connectivity, with its implicit urgency, through your phone and computer encourages the adrenal glands to produce stress hormones which can temporally boost energy levels but as a long-standing living condition can lead to disassociation on an emotional level and eventual impairment of memory and brain function.[10] Time out from this connectivity needs to be part of 'taking more time for yourself'.

It can also be all too easy to unwittingly keep your nervous energy up to mark, especially over any difficult period in your career, with a regular diet of chocolate digestives or

---

[10] Research by Dr Gary Small, UCLA. More information at: http://newsroom.ucla.edu/stories/081015_gary-small-ibrain. Quoted in M. Harris (2014) *The End of Absence*, Penguin (pertinent and worth reading).

whatever is your preferred sugar fix. I speak as one with a hand that regularly hovers over the cookie jar.

In order to move seamlessly from the everyday to your work mode, choose to take some moments to stop and think yourself upwards, as your Alexander teacher shows you, before you travel to performance, rehearsal or read through. This helps prevent any head retraction and contraction of neck muscles and enlivens your energy. Before you arrive at the venue you will already be 'tuned up' ready to go.

Dem Bones

Your toe bone connected to your foot bone
Your foot bone connected to your ankle bone
Your ankle bone connected to your leg bone
Your leg bone connected to your knee bone
Your knee bone connected to your thigh bone
Your thigh bone connected to your hip bone
Your hip bone connected to your back bone
Your back bone connected to your shoulder bone
Your shoulder bone connected to your neck bone
Your neck bone connected to your head bone[11]

Making the parts work for you (as a whole)

As the song has it, everything in the body connects up. Those muscles that appear to be behaving independently of each other connect in beautiful spiralling patterns when you are moving. In turn they exert little pulls on the skeletal system, the bones they are attached to, and the joints, all the time.

It is useful to make a quick check through the body to identify where the essentials are really located. But before that, a word. Images are seldom evoked[12] when applying the Alexander technique. Here's one reason why: the great American dancer, Martha Graham, a pioneer of modern dance, taught that her movement comes from the pelvis as a contraction and release but she recognised the immensely important role the back plays in doing the actual work.

---

[11] 'Dem Bones' written by James Weldon Johnson.

[12] For some people visualisation is impossible: a condition called aphantasia. Using thought instead may help to bypass this situation.

In London during a pre-performance speech (at an advanced age, regally resplendent, seated on an impressive stage throne) I heard her talk about the wonderful snake in the body, the spine. When you imagine yours as a snake you base that image on your *experience* of your spine. If, as you will have noted, it's all too easy to regularly stiffen your neck and pull down into your back then that's the memory you will use, of a rather tame and short snake.

Most of us forget that the spine starts in the middle of the head (not in the neck) where the head is supported on the atlanto-occipital joint which allows for a very small movement back and forth only. If you move your fingers round from the hollow under both ears to the tip of your nose that is the level of the joint (which can't be felt from the outside). From there all the way to the end of the tail bone can make, after all, for a rather lithesome splendid snake. By paying attention to the lively dynamic of the head-neck-back rather than the use of image, the spine finds the space it needs, without any faulty judgement, to retain the length it is designed to have.

In a four-footed animal it is easy to see how important the spine is as most of the inner organs are, for want of a better phrase, slung from it. Although we are in the upright we are in a similar state of dependence. Our various life systems and organs expect the spine to be long and mobile in order to accommodate optimum functioning. So everything is connected and reliant on the 'back bone'.

The picture we can often carry around of our own skeleton is based on the bones we see (in exhibitions and pictures, butcher blocks and dog bowls), that are no longer designated for living use.

It is easy to be unaware of bone's extraordinary properties of elasticity and connections to the tides of activity in the body.[13] The animated springiness of our approximately 206

---

13 See an article in the *New York Times* by Natalie Angier: https://www.nytimes.com/2009/04/28/science/28angi.html

bones is supported by a constant input from signalling molecules, hormones and a form of on-the-spot bone remodelling, at any given point, simultaneously, in the structure of a bone. All this to maintain flexibility and adaptability for your multi-tasking system. For, at the same time as a healthy skeleton allows you to be fully mobile, it also houses marrow for the production of blood cells and provides calcium for many biochemical needs.

Along with a French colleague I used to give Alexander technique themed holidays (in France, Ireland and the UK). Marie-Claude Maisonneuve would ask us all to take time together to reflect silently on the skeleton. At the time we giggled and thought she was being rather extreme but soon realised the wisdom of that exercise. Familiarising myself with... myself!

Having an increased sense of the aliveness of your body's own framework joins up all the dots and, even without being a trained dancer, encourages a holistic and integrated gracefulness from head turn to ankle swivel.

The articulated areas of the skeleton and surrounding muscles can be particularly susceptible to the effects of perceived stress. The jaw joint is quick to tighten. Sometimes it's difficult to change that. There is tasty advice, however, from Alexander teacher and dentist Barry Collins, to retain (in your mind) a marshmallow between your back teeth, which instantly frees up the space. Notice what else is going on. Are you holding your breath? It often happens when listening to someone speak. Where is your tongue? Sometimes it can become clamped up tensely to the roof of your mouth. Unless you have a very good reason for doing so, it is much better to let it rest in between times, at the bottom of your mouth. Its strong root is behind the voice box and connects and pulls on all the muscles around it.

A bone not talked about very much outside cranio-sacral and osteopathic circles, is the sphenoid bone. It is situated in the middle of the skull as though behind the eyes and is also known as the butterfly bone (as it resembles a butterfly with wings extended). Deeply embedded, it strongly affects all the bones of the cranium. The work of Dr. Viola Frymann, D.O. showed that it is not only adversely affected by head and neck trauma but continually responds to your vocalising, chewing and even, with a tiny flutter of its wings, to your breathing. Life as it is lived doesn't encourage you to think of yourself as a delicate balancing mechanism with unseen sensitive components. Retain awareness of this inherent fragile equilibrium, it contributes to the refined sensitivity in your life and art.

The head can remain poised while you open your mouth. One of the signs of a nervous (or unaware) actor in performance is that tipping of the head back onto the spine while pulling in a preliminary breath through the mouth. Before rehearsing your lines or a prepared speech remember your teacher's calm hand, and practise using your thought to direct your neck to be free so you can allow the tip (only) of the nose to drop 1 cm or ¼ of an inch (as in a secret or practically invisible 'yes') at the same time as you open your mouth. This quickly takes any unnecessary pressure off the spine and prevents your head kicking backwards. Your head weighs about six kilos – a fearsome amount to be pressing down on the neck and spine.

Beware of the 'just in case' nod – a misinterpretation of the previous instruction where, ignoring the location of the joint, the head hangs down from the middle of the neck.

With awareness, you can of course move your head however you like without tightening the neck. You do not need to go round like the dog in the back of the car window visibly nodding when still, moving or speaking. You are, however, conscious of the available freedom.

"Leg bone connected to your knee bone." It is very easy to overextend the legs by pushing the knees backwards. It can give a feeling of solidity and being 'grounded' but I am afraid this is another illusion. Knees also need the wobble factor.

Now you don't have to go around in demi-plié but they should be ready to go downhill skiing at any time. Remember when they instead become clenched and the legs stiffened there is a direct effect all the way through the torso. It's such a strong and mostly[14] unnecessary habit for many people, so please don't distress yourself if you keep noticing it happening. The important thing is that you have noticed. Allow the release and then don't worry. It can change!

Singing in a folk group in The Netherlands in the 1980s I was so nervous performing that my legs would shake. I automatically gripped to stop it showing, little realising at the time that this habit was making it more difficult for me to breathe and sing.

Hip joints are not at the bony pelvic girdle that holds up your trousers, but lower down. Dig your fingers into the top of your legs and walk on the spot and you will feel them working. It is essential that you know their location. Bending to lift a heavy object, you do not want to lower from the waist as, unlike the hips, it is not a joint designed to bear weight. That is the way to back strain.

Your sitting bones are designed for... sitting upon. Modern chairs and manners make it easy to sit instead on your tail bone. Small and easily weakened, compressing it to take your weight also causes the loss of the lower curve of your spine which in turn affects the functioning of the diaphragm.

To rediscover your seat bones, sit on the edge of a chair with both feet on the ground. Slip your hands under your bottom and feel the bones there... that's them.

Like rockers they can tilt you forward onto your thighs or backwards towards your tail. Sitting on a seat that slopes forward (try paperback books under the back legs of a four-legged chair) frees up your hip joints and makes it more

---

14 Those with a tendency to hypermobility may find it feels necessary to remain upright without discomfort. It will soon become clear if that is the case or is in fact a changeable habit.

comfortable to experience sitting on your seat bones and let your spine be long. You actually need to find them to successfully balance sitting on a large blow up ball. On horseback you also need to be in contact with sitting bones to communicate adequately and be settled on your horse.

The remnants of a received notion of military uprightness as being the best model lingers in the admonition to straighten up and pull the shoulders back and down. This 'correct position' for shoulders narrows the upper back, contracts the torso and is difficult to maintain for very long. It certainly doesn't make for easy breath or speech. It is still, however, in the background of the instruction to 'do something' about tight, rounded or raised shoulders. Remember the surrounding muscles will take time to adjust and release as you allow expansion in the torso. Don't ever think of them as a problem but as a linked-up part of your arm and back support network. Imbue your shoulders with a new soft personality and remind them that they are designed to float away from each other and do not have to have undue responsibility for the weight of the arms.

Your arms are like wings. The muscle attachments go into the neck and the back. As with wings, the feathers need time to unruffle. Letting your arms rest on your lap, palms upward, is a kind gift to them from time to time (this also prevents the shoulders from automatically sloping forwards and down). Arms work hard during the day and often when you think they are 'relaxed' they are carrying some residual tension. If they were over-engaged when you drove to rehearsal or carried a heavy bag, the activity will inform your gesture and balance in the run through. It is not being precious to pay great attention to how you are using your arms in ordinary activity as much as the more obvious components of the free body and easy voice. When you take time for some Alexander lying down and let your hands rest on your torso, notice those wing-like connections and let their weight fall heavily down through your elbows into the floor.

The heel bones are under the ankle joints and are my favourite bones in the body. Designed to take a considerable amount of body weight, I firmly believe they are an actor's best friend as I expound in other chapters.

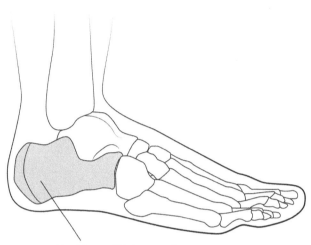

Heel bone ('Calcaneus')

A Generous Voice

Smelling a beautiful flower, it's unlikely that you sniff or gasp. With the delicate scent wafting gently into your nostrils the air passageways open spontaneously and your lungs fill up easily while your tummy muscles relax. Hmmm. On a visit to Rodin's garden in Paris there were the most delicious sherbety smelling old roses, I can still recall the scent.

Smell a rose in passing and notice what happens to your body!

This is the model for a practical natural inhalation through the nose where the air is filtered and warmed before it reaches the lungs.[15] However you choose to use your breath in performance, this is the foundation for your everyday breathing and the starting point for any breathing technique you may learn.

Rather than 'taking a deep breath', which easily creates fixedness in the torso, imagine into action gently smelling a sweet-scented flower. It is what you can come back to when you feel stage fright, stress, uncertainty or imbalance. Close the mouth and the breath will come in quite quickly through the nose and if your back has adequate length you will have enough space for the expanding movement of the ribs.

If up to now you have become used to breathing mostly through the mouth it takes time to trust this. The point isn't that you must always breathe in through your nose but that you can have the choice to do so or not when it suits. When you breathe out or vocalise, ribs swing inwards following the contraction of the lungs as they empty, but at no point does the upper chest need to sink down. The direction you are

---

[15] See Elaine Morgan (1994) *The Scars of Evolution,* Souvenir Press Ch. 11.

going in is still 'up'. This is easy to remember as your voice floats out upwards from your mouth so you can allow your spine to maintain the 'strength of its length' in both exhalation and inhalation. Pressing down into the chest or abdomen does nothing to increase breath span or embellish vocal tone.

A reminder here that the spine runs through the centre of the body, not only where you can feel the bony vertebrae. This is why a disturbance in the spine can sometimes also be felt in the front of your body. As all the muscles in the body run in spirals and connect to each other in the muscular chain when you move, if – as I did – you find yourself nervously tightening up your legs, knees braced back, you can expect corresponding tightness in and around the armpits. This stops the easy rib swing and breath flow, just when it is most needed. Over-tensing and pulling down both interfere with vocal production and especially the free functioning of the diaphragm. You speak with your whole self, so how you are thinking (as you have already found) and what you are doing with all sorts of odd parts of the body will have an effect on the whole of you, including every aspect of utterance. The vocal mechanism (the voice box) is suspended in musculature that is attached to the head. When the head is supported in balance (on the atlanto-occipital joint) there is no need for pull or strain in the throat.

The diaphragm is an often-misunderstood muscle. It is like a gentle giant in the body, quietly ensuring breathing action. You do not have to do anything to get it to work; it will do it all for you. Some of the exercise work you do on strengthening breath control via the diaphragm is actually focusing on the abdominal muscles (including the transverse abdominis) which will then do a different job. Please note that, despite popular thinking, these muscles cannot be trained in isolation from other muscles nor, studies show, do they normally give the spine essential support.[16]

As it is a muscle over which we do not have direct control (an involuntary muscle) you either interfere with the workings of the gentle giant or you leave it alone to get on with things and simply ensure it can work as easily as possible.

An anchoring tendon attachment for the diaphragm is an insertion at the front of the lower part of the spine in the lumbar curve. If this curve is unnaturally over-extended or collapsed while you are speaking or singing it cannot function so efficiently. A release of tension in the legs and the buttocks allows the root of the diaphragm to operate without interference.

In simple terms, at a given signal from the brain, the diaphragm wants to expand to tickle the ribs reminding them to open out for inhalation. It goes back to its resting position during exhalation.

Breathing however is 'on the wheel'. As the breath exits there is already an in-breath imperceptibly beginning – Nature doesn't usually like a vacuum.

Except in extreme cases of illness you don't have to 'do' the action. Sometimes the breathing and vocal techniques you may learn for performance call on your strong use of the abdominal muscles. It is important to remember, again, that this is not every day breathing and just like the actor playing Quasimodo you do not want to bring the hump to breakfast. Regularly depending on a forceful way of using your breath and muscles in normal conversation develops a habitual and restricting tension which will eventually impede the full depth and breadth of the voice.[17]

Surprisingly, opening the mouth is fraught with hazards.

---

16 Thanks to Dr Miriam Wohl for pointing me to Eyal Lederman's 'Myth of Core Stability': www.cpdo.net/ Lederman_The_myth_of_core_stability.pdf

17 For an excellent description of voice production, see the chapter 'About Breathing' in Elizabeth Langford (2008) *Mind and Muscle, an owner's handbook*, Garant Uitgevers.

The habit of tilting the head backwards in order to open the mouth, instead of only allowing the jaw to gently slide open, not only looks awful in a performer it pulls on the muscles in the throat and tenses the neck muscles.

Smoking cigarettes regularly predisposes the smoker to an established habit of sucking breath in through the mouth, unnecessarily contracting throat muscles, preparatory to speaking. You don't have to be a smoker of course to have this habit. Many public or media figures display a similar muscle tightening action in conversation and speechifying and this can disconcertingly create tension in the listener in unconscious imitation.

Get back to smelling the flowers! Watching a shoal of sardines going round and round in an aquarium in San Francisco I was struck by the free movement of their opening mouths as they trawled for any passing food. This, I thought, is how easily the mouth is designed to open either for eating or utterance! A decision to stop (momentarily), before you open your mouth to sing or speak and to direct your thought to free your neck, as learned in your Alexander lessons, not only avoids strain and interference but also consequently enriches the tone and expression of the voice. Practise opening your mouth as freely as a hungry fish but if you can, rather than looking hang-dog, keep your eyes bright and alive at the same time, maybe looking out for smaller fish...

Eye muscles also have habits and can become very shy when you are speaking or even breathing in during a pause in performance or public speaking. It is quite helpful to take on the habit of looking out at an imagined audience when you are breathing between lines 'in rehearsal' at home. You can even try taking the time to allow the breath to come in through the nose and find it suits the rhythm of the writing. Rather than it being your head that 'looks', let the eyes begin the movement when moving the head from side to side and up and down. Then you are less likely to appear as though you have no neck at all. This 'no neck' phenomenon is quite prevalent and lessens the ability to move freely and in whatever style best suits a role.

One of the advantages of awareness of the Alexander principles when opening the mouth and speaking is this consequent freeing and gentle lengthening of the neck. The voice box finds itself close to the spine and its vibration is felt in the bones. Sometimes singers and speakers use this awareness to speak out of the back of their heads, as it were.

Resonance is something you are used to exploiting through the bones and cavities in the head, face, neck and in the chest but it is exciting to realise that if the spine and larynx are in close proximity the vibration of the voice is carried throughout the body by the skeletal system and the entire organism can become a sounding board for the voice. Speaking with the whole self becomes a practical reality. Even your feet can tingle with the sound you make.

Another factor to consider in this equation is that the sound of your voice with its attending vibration actually has health-giving qualities, for you! Alfred Tomatis, the eminent French Ear Nose and Throat doctor, confirmed the energy-giving properties of the voice in the following case. In 1966 when the 4-hourly regular chanting, which had been practised by monks all their monastic lives, was discontinued in one abbey, the monks all fell ill and listless. After many months of other medical interventions Professor Tomatis was eventually consulted and his diagnosis proved correct. It was only when the chanting was finally resumed that full health could return to the community.[18]

The monks made sure to connect with their sitting bones when standing chanting. They balanced, from time to time, on the misericord, a small promontory on the underside of their hinged seats (still to be found in old churches especially the choir stalls) to monitor and utilise this bone conduction to support their voices (and consequently their energy).

---

[18] A.A. Tomatis (1991) *The Conscious Ear*, Station Hill Press

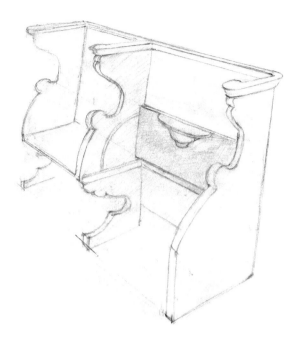

A major energising factor of performance is when you use your voice in its full capacity, without restriction. The vibration of the free voice relayed through bone conduction is a strong stimulus to the vagus nerve which tracks through the body delivering to the various organs its vibratory information like a splendid postal system. Vagus, aptly, is Latin for wandering.

The connectedness to an audience, the refined interaction with a fellow player, adrenaline and the effects of applause (described by Mrs Jordan in 1810 as "internal exultation, a delight bordering on ecstasy") all contribute to the 'high' after performance.[19] A lasting heightened sense of 'aliveness' is often, however, particularly due to effects of the inner

---

[19] Mrs Jordan is quoted in Claire Tomalin's *Mrs Jordan's Profession* (1995). Laurence Olivier described the thrill of acting in front of an audience as like 'Coming for a living' (as in having orgasms) – quoted in Tarquin Olivier's book *My Father Laurence Olivier.*

reaches of the free voice.

There are voices that please and voices that do not. A grounded voice with a thoughtful connection to the feet (especially the heel bones) gives the voice somewhere to soar from. A neck free of tension will allow vibrational resonance to occur throughout the body.

Producing sound also makes the outside air vibrate. To listen to someone else singing or speaking is to enter into a 'partnership of vibration'. Listeners who are situated in this air space will find themselves 'sculpted' by the vibrations. When you are using yourself and your voice well you can lift your audience and even inspire and brighten them with your generous voice. If you are breathing with ease, then they can as well and will be more receptive to your performance. The converse of course is also true.

If you didn't already have enough to think about, I am now suggesting your audience's wellbeing is in your hands, or your throat.[20] In 1986 I attended a West End matinee of 'Mr and Mrs Nobody' by Keith Waterhouse, with Judi Dench and her late husband Michael Williams in the title roles. We were a dismal little audience of about 14 on a wet afternoon in London. I would have forgiven the actors for coming to our level and giving us a fair to average performance. I have never forgotten, however, the impact Judi Dench's energy had on me. Her voice didn't scold, didn't urge me to sit up in my seat, her presence wasn't strident, but she was committed to the performance and drew the whole audience into an energised state to match her own. That is what she did: she brought us up to her level. However she did it, whatever skills, techniques and marvellous intuition she used, it worked and sent us all out into the rain in a much better state than when we had arrived.

---

[20] See my paper 'The Generous Voice' (1994) which was given to the International Congress of Alexander Teachers, Oxford and is online at: www.alexandertec.net and at www.triarchypress.net/generous

Conversations with Alex

Over several years, the voice teacher Alex Bingley and I have exchanged ideas about the role the Alexander technique can play in supporting voice and text work for actors. In his teaching he has developed quite an extensive connection between his own experience of Alexander principles and what is helpful for performers. He continues his research with the work of Alexander teachers Nadia Kevan & Ron Murdock.

Working together, some of the conclusions we came to are quite simple but in class and rehearsal we have both found them effective. Here are a few of them for you to enjoy.

Sounds with Ribs

While you are lying down in the Alexander constructive rest position (see page 56) your breathing becomes quieter, is more calm and easy. Notice the ribs pressing into the ground and allow the air to come in gently through the nose. Using sustained vowel sounds (and continuing to note the movement of the ribs) utter them without concern for their duration but close the mouth when finished so the air can come in gently through the nose.

Sitting

If seated for voice work, change the habitual sitting pattern by sitting on the edge and tilting (safely) a chair forward while your feet are firmly on the ground. This ensures a connection to the sitting bones (remember the misericord used by the monks) and frees up the hips and legs. When sitting on the floor for any length of time, having a firm cushion, bag or books to sit on takes the strain off the hip joints and the lower back. Sitting on a table with feet dangling also shifts the usual dynamic.

Running to Speak

Instead of preparing with a special breath, stop for a moment to remember your head poise before running around the space gently singing an Ah sound on one breath. Stop and stand still, connecting to your heel bones, just before you 'run out of breath', speak a few words and discover that there is, after all, breath available. Experiment to see how much breath you really need to speak a line.

The Floating Breath

To appreciate the potential of a small, short, fragile breath, imagine a feather in front of your mouth that you keep afloat with your delicate breath. Then, with the same thought, sing a very soft Ah, allowing only the movement of the ribs to sustain the sound.

On Hands and Knees

To vocalise when crawling, let the crown of the head lead (not head hanging or face looking up) while the spine lengthens towards the tail of the spine. Play with cross patterning using all four limbs on the diagonal – hand and opposite knee – as a cat walks (or as babies often move around).

And a special thought: in one exchange, Alex told me that he was reminded that the Greek root of the name xiphoid, the process or extension which projects downwards from the sternum, means *sword like* (it looks like the tip of a sword blade) and this is what protects our hearts.[21] Our heart, he says, does need protection so that we are not overwhelmed by the world; but it made him think that when we are holding too tightly it might be harder to speak or sing from the heart.

---

[21] In fact, projecting downward from the point where the lowermost ribs join the sternum "the xiphoid process functions as a vital attachment point for several major muscles. It acts as one of several origins for the diaphragm muscle that forms the floor of the ribcage. The xiphoid process also acts as an insertion for the rectus abdominis and transverse abdominis muscles that compress and flex the abdomen". [Tim Taylor, anatomy and physiology instructor, www.innerbody.com]

The Slow Bicycle Race

In 1931 when my mother was at school, the slow bicycle race was well known. The idea of a 'race' where the winner finishes last is fun, but unfortunately is no longer a regular fixture in sports departments.

It is, however, an excellent sport in which to excel as the only way to win this competition and not fall off the bicycle is to first have a mastery over your own balance. Unlike a horse, the bicycle cannot 'right' itself however the rider behaves.

Slowing things right down can often make it awkward to retain equilibrium. I once watched brave English National Opera Chorus singers wobbling their way in slow motion across the stage during a preview performance of the original 1985 English National Opera's production of Philip Glass's Opera, 'Akhnaten'.

It appeared that, perhaps being under-rehearsed, little instruction had been given as to how they were going to achieve this 'unnatural' gait while all the time gallantly continuing to sing.

In your normal, everyday way of moving you may lean, lurch and slide yourself around without paying any heed to your balance. Without conscious awareness, however, and confronted with a sloping surface, steps, uneven ground on or off the stage or the differing physical demands of a character, you can easily hurt yourself. When you are tired and pulling yourself downwards, you are also more likely to go over on your ankle if a paving stone is uneven, (I know, it's happened to me). Many people in Western society walk by putting a foot forward to stop themselves falling. This doesn't leave very much margin for error. If this is your normal way of getting around you will be quite put out when asked to slow it down or change it, tottering, unsteady on the feet.

Any of us who attempt jogging or running will relate to the experience some athletes recount that at a certain point in a race the brain wants one thing and the body another, and that they have to override the mind's inclination to stop, and keep the feet moving in the race. This is helped by developing a comfortable familiarity with what the feet are supposed to be 'doing' at any given time. Refreshing your acquaintance with your feet by feeling them spread out over the ground and giving them time to feel the earth as you move increases your appreciation of their reliability. More inspiringly, the creative funambulist Philippe Petit, who should know, writes about trusting the gods in his feet in *To Reach the Clouds*.

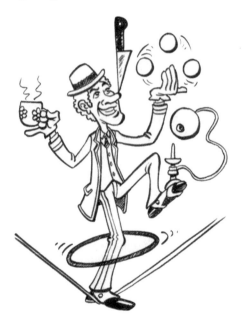

When balancing in everyday walking I like to think of the feet as our mobile anchors, our connection to the earth and the spring point for when I choose to defy gravity.

First of all, you have to accept that you are balancing on a rotating planet and that, whether you know it or not, you are never standing still. Even when you think you are, your system is making minute adjustments all the time, not only to the progress of circulating fluids in your own body but also to the changes beneath your feet. Gravity maintains your connection to the earth without you having to think about it and, when you take on responsibility for ensuring the freedom of your joints and 'uprightness', the bonus is that you also recover the ability to balance with much less effort.

When walking, it is necessary to allow yourself the possibility of being slightly off balance in motion in order to retain a continually adjusting equilibrium integrating the inherent small wobble with ease. Every step can seem like a leap in faith when thought about in this way. We are designed, however, to be able to walk and balance on one foot after the other without falling downwards – a gentle dance on the tightrope of life. Even with four feet a cat's front paws are light on the ground or hover above it until sure of the suitability of the terrain. Feel the whole foot working as you walk. Notice the heel strike, the slight roll and the connection to the toes especially the big toe as you launch off to the next step. Because weight is going down, you have somewhere to come up from.

To balance within your own upright stature, use the reference point of 60% of your weight being taken by your heel bone (under the ankle joint) and 40% through the ball of the foot at the big and little toes (incidentally now your head can find its balancing point more easily). Barefoot or in flat shoes play with this swaying backwards and forwards, never so far that your toes or heels come off the ground. Experiment anywhere with this redistribution of weight bearing: at the bus stop, waiting for the kettle to boil. Become used to the freedom of your ankles so that with this thought you are less likely to automatically tip forward as you speak, extend a hand or move.

It is possible that before now the ratio was reversed so do not worry if it feels uncomfortable at first. Wearing high heels places quite extreme demands on the feet. If you often wear them your muscles may need time to adjust to the new way of balancing. Do not force the issue but keep reminding yourself of the new possibility. It's helpful to alternate footwear daily and when not medically necessary to avoid regularly wearing shoes with inbuilt arch supports. The arch is the spring of the foot that wants to work to support you. Let it do its job!

When in doubt about lines, breath, freeing the neck, or being heard when you are shouting for someone's attention, think of your connection to your heel bones. You may find yourself imperceptibly moving back through the ankles towards them but don't push yourself in that direction... the toes still have to remain earthbound!

Planting your feet in a position is not 'grounding' yourself. If you find you have done so, gently adjust their position to what may feel slightly unfamiliar (good!) and become accustomed to not minding any 'uncertainty' about balancing on two legs.

It is very likely however that women especially will wear heels from time to time in performance. If this is the case it is essential that you practise consciously in them as often as possible with great awareness of the adjustments you need to make, to avoid unnecessary tightening of ankles and neck and throat, etc.

In Los Angeles, my friend Stephanie Silverman played the part of a vulture. She wore treacherous spike heels and was the hit of the show but only because "I practiced over and over in the heels to be able to at one point perch on a tiny platform and slowly turn completely around".

Choosing to anticipate and accustom yourself *over time* to a slope, high heels, ladders, steps, anything that isn't the expected flat playing area, gives you the flexibility to quickly adapt when called to.

It may seem logical that, when gesturing with an arm or picking up an object in front of you, you go forwards to do so. The opposite is much more helpful. Practise swaying and notice that as soon as you go further towards the toes it's very likely that your head tilts backwards to stop you falling.

Instead as you lift your arm let yourself come backwards, ever so slightly, through the ankles to counterbalance the weight of your arm (heavier than you think). This way you will not disturb the freedom you need in your body, to move fluidly and speak clearly.

Watching birds, seemingly at play, riding the thermals over the lake in Québec, where I am writing this book, I am struck by how they are balancing in the air, without effort, using the environment to keep them afloat. Earth-bound creatures can also find a lively support, from the ground beneath us. [22] We also need contact with our feet or our sitting bones in order to balance and to have somewhere to go up from.

Keeping awareness of what is going on around you, take a walk while thinking (only) of the weight being on the back foot rather than the front foot and notice any difference it makes. At risk of becoming part of Monty Python's Ministry of Silly Walks, every now and then stop 'mid walk' and keep one foot poised off the ground to remind yourself that you are walking on one foot after the other. Don't hold your breath at the same time! If you have a bicycle why not (although never on a public thoroughfare!) emulate your child self; keep your Alexander directions in mind and try having a nice slow wobble.

---

[22] Having written this sentence based on my own experience of 'ground support', I came across Nadia Kevan's chapter 'The Vitality and Grace of the Performing Artist' in Claire Rennie et al. (2015) *Connected Perspectives*, Hite Books. In it she talks of her study of indigenous tribes and how "They stand firmly on the ground. Their strength, energy and radiance seems to rise up out of the ground through their feet..."

The Thinking Spine

"I want to see back acting – Italian back acting", is something my friend Ivan Midderigh of the Roy Hart theatre often demands of his students as a way to encourage a more enlivened expression. Focusing on what is in front of you, showing your face to the world, can be a primary occupation of the performer. Even your ribs may suspend their potential back expansion causing you to become quite two dimensional as you engage with the audience.

"Be careful dear boy, I have just walked there", reportedly Laurence Olivier's remark to a young actor during rehearsal, might not have been an ego gone mad but rather an awareness of the sizzling quality of the energy he generated all around him which included the full involvement of the power of his back.

Looking after your back is essential to good health but perhaps for the performer there is another exciting reason to maintain the best use of your spine. It is charming to realise that, like the writing in an old-fashioned stick of souvenir seaside rock, there is a shape embedded throughout the spinal cord – a butterfly. It encloses grey matter similar to that found in the brain. As well as processing and editing billions of incoming stimuli before passing the information on to the brain, it contributes directly to our spatial awareness in movement and self-awareness in relation to gravity and 'groundedness'.

Although the spinal cord is not the brain per se (and unlike the Stegosaurus we are not suspected of having one at either end of the spine), it may be that the information it receives and the way the spinal cord synthesises those incoming messages 'lays the foundations for conscious thought'. These are cornerstones for an accumulation of untouched sub-verbal ideas that feed your impulse to bring forward something completely different in role, understanding or life.

The late Sam Shepard, when talking about creating characters in his plays, said "I mean you have these assumptions about somebody and all of a sudden this other thing appears. Where is that coming from? That's the mystery, that's what's so fascinating."

If, as I believe, the major source of creativity and inspiration is in an interaction with the unexplored and the unknown, the unexplained and the unconscious, then it is pretty certain this connection is never found in personal patterns of habit. Preventing the habitual reaction can be a gift, a space for the unexpected and truly creative to emerge.

So, in looking after your thinking sensitive spine in all its lovely bendy strength, you could be nurturing and accommodating your next great idea, inspired characterisation or witty remark.

Sometimes a sudden backache or worse can occur after receiving an emotional shock (not only from a physical straining or an accident). In a study of the effects of psychological stress during lifting it was found that mental processes/stress had a large impact on the spine.[23]

This sensibility means your spine is quite attuned to your feelings and it is important, as some Alexander technique teachers are fond of reminding you, to 'listen' to your back. Take great care not to try and override the discomfort without taking due note of what you need at that time, whether it is sleep, space, quiet or some outside help.

This paying attention or listening is not based on whimsical conceit. Along with the contribution of thought it has practical application. In an illuminating essay, Pam Walatka quotes a Californian professor of spinal cord injury

---

[23] See Eyal Lederman's 'Myth of Core Stability' (2014):
www.cpdo.net/Lederman_The_myth_of_core_stability.pdf

at Stanford University: "The idea of a mind in the spinal cord does make sense to me in light of my experience with spinal cord injury patients. My patients learn to use the mind in their spinal cords to improve musculo-skeletal function."[24]

Usually without serious injury to contend with, Alexander teachers and students experience using conscious thought to improve many elements in their functioning in all everyday activities including encouraging a lengthening of the back.

An input of directed thought ensures the spine has the space to be the length it wants to be. When you initiate this kind of contact and then take the time to 'listen' to your spine you can unexpectedly find the means to uncover your own creative goldmine.

Probably inspired by the massive whale bones still on view in his studio in Perry Green, Hertfordshire, Henry Moore's giant sculpture of vertebrae magnifies the fantastic durability and strength of the spine as well as its beauty.

More recently the Derry born artist Eilis O' Connell depicts it as a 'body and soul circuit' evoking many delicate, imaginative, refined qualities that you can find deeply embedded in your own being.

Not taking any part of your capacity or talent for granted means changing your perception. Recognise that your spine is the patient mainstay of your creative output. Then your 'back acting' could really become something to watch out for.

The following lifetime's homework looks after your back, and as an actor pupil said: "It gives you a second chance when you've goofed up during the day".

---

[24] 'The Mind in the Spine' an essay by Pam Walatka:
http://pamsyogafitness.com/articles/the-mind-in-the-spine.shtml.
See also recent research about the 'mini brain' in the spine carried out by the Salk Institute, La Jolla California and described here:
www.salk.edu/news-release/walking-on-ice-takes-more-than-brains/

Alexander Lying Down

This is an excellent practice for pre-performance or any time. For up to 20 minutes, when you can, lie on the floor. Stay in quietness or listen to music or the spoken word, paying attention to yourself from time to time.

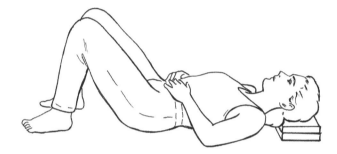

Lie down with your head (not your neck) on books and let your knees come up, (without tensing your neck). Your feet are on the ground and your hands are (unclasped) resting on your tummy or hips. Your eyes remain open and you are alert. A good guide for the height of books you need is to measure the span of your hand from the base of the little finger to that of the thumb. However, be comfortable and use less or more as you wish. Be aware of the points where you are being supported: your head on the books, shoulder area, elbows, hip area and two feet. Think of sending your knees up to the ceiling and directing any weight down through the feet at the ball of the foot at the big toe, even if it's not where you feel the weight. If there is a little arch in the lower back, there is no need to try to flatten it to the floor. When muscle is over-contracted there it will usually release in its own time (today, tomorrow, next week). Nor is it any help to try to push the shoulders back. Leave them alone. You can think of the points of the shoulders floating away from each other if you like. Notice how your arm is wing-like. Note the outside of the hand and outside of the arm connecting into your back. Let the weight of the busy and heavy arm fall down through the elbow. There are a lot of muscle insertions in the armpits which can easily become over-tensed. When you are lying down, gravity will help your spine to lengthen and allow a 'widening' to happen, a spreading as it were, from upper arm to upper arm which includes addressing any contraction in the arm pits. With the head already 'forward and up' on the books and without having to support the weight of the head, your neck can more easily be free from holding.

Think of sending your head away from your feet, the whole back/torso to lengthen and widen, (ensure you are not holding on behind the knees). Directing at intervals, while you are lying down, reinforces the experience of an Alexander lesson and helps your system to respond to similar directed thoughts when you are in the upright. Asking for widening from upper arm to upper arm also gives space for the ribs to move freely.

When coming to standing from lying down (and getting out of bed in the morning), let your head gently roll in the direction you are going to get up, to let it lead the movement.

This exercise has become known as semi-supine (half of supine) which describes what it looks like as a useful position for recovery and relaxed preparation; but without the above awareness it remains only that. I prefer to call it 'constructive rest', 'active lying down' or plain 'Alexander lying down'!

Although not a 'sleeping period' this conscious exercise also allows for what Thierry Paquot calls a "brief interval to take our bearings, just as the sailor marks his position and plots his course while all around him the elements either rage or subside."[25]

---

[25] Thierry Paquot (2005) *The Art of the Siesta*, Marion Boyars.

Unhelpful Stress

When you are feeling worried or insufficiently relaxed, a popular method of addressing tension is to focus on an unrelaxed part of the body, deliberately tensing muscle and then 'letting it go'. This brings a feeling of relief.

The exaggerated over-holding and then relaxing feels as though the problem is addressed. In reality, however, it takes a split second to contract muscle and a lot longer for that same muscle to de-contract or 'release'. In other words, this action is compounding the original difficulty of over-tensed muscle for the sake of a fleeting feeling of relief based on an inaccurate sensory perception.

There are often unnoticed tensions that won't even be addressed by this method. During my acting training, I was once ill-advisedly told to send any stress to my feet. Depending on your footwear you may be doing this anyway by stiffening your feet to shuffle about in those indoor slippers or curling your toes tight to keep a pair of unsecured shoes from slipping off.

As an actor you are used to evaluating the impact of thought processes on development of role and characterisation. When confronted with unhelpful stress and tension what you need is to get in behind those thought processes and examine your attitude, to separate the activity or thought from the emotional additive.

You are likely to notice what happens to you when you do become stressed and what brings it about. For myself I note that my jaw becomes held and I have a tendency to over-organise both myself and other people when I have not had enough space or time to myself. It is important to acknowledge what are the most difficult scenarios for you and to differentiate between unhelpful and useful 'stress' – that challenge which stretches you beyond your imagined limit. Being very busy and in demand (or however you become out of sorts) doesn't mean you have to also feel stressed.

It all depends on your attitude.

In most situations you can make a choice as to how you are going to respond mentally/emotionally and indeed practically. It's at this point, however, that the old unconscious habits can, instead, kick in (my tightened jaw). The idea of a quick fix, tensing and releasing, can seem very appealing. In your Alexander lessons you learn to use your mind to bring about release in habitually over-contracted muscles. Not through an action but through using your thought in a structured manner to free yourself in an upward direction. You remember that this procedure primarily begins with a wish to release muscles held in the neck. You learn to think of yourself as a whole, where inappropriate muscle tension in one area has consequences for the whole balancing mechanism. Paying attention to the process of shedding tension ensures an equally holistic and quality result!

Eva Tanguay[26], the original 'I don't care' girl, sang:

> I don't care, I don't care,
> If people don't like me,
> I'll try to outlive it,
> I know I'll forgive it,
> And live contentedly.
> I don't care, I don't care,

---

[26] Eva Tanguay was reputedly one of the highest paid performers in 1910 ($3,500 per week). (Thank you to Kent Baker for telling me about her and for singing me the song) The extract is from 'I don't care', words by Jean Lenox, music by Harry Sutton. Published (1905) by Jerome H. Remick.

If people do not try to treat me fair.
There is naught can amaze me,
Dislike cannot daze me,
'Cos I don't care.

Worry involves a physical demonstration of emotion, a furrowing of the brow, a holding of the breath, a jigging of a leg or a tensing of any part of the anatomy.

Some time ago I noticed on waking up in the morning that my tongue was tightened against the roof of my mouth so I realised I was quite bothered about an issue. One way to help the technique work effectively for you is to make the decision that rather than worry about something you will only think about it instead. I could take a step back from the problem and find some constructive resolution which let my tongue relax while I slept. You could also cultivate an 'I don't care' attitude (as exemplified in the song). This isn't to encourage you to be an uncaring or irresponsible person but to remind you of the small difference in approach that gives you a space to make clearer choices.

Withdrawal from habitual mental over-involvement is echoed in the physical awareness that you have about balance and freedom in your poise and movement. Being regularly forward on your toes when out of the dance arena might be an indication that you are already hastily in the next moment without fully appreciating yourself and all possibilities in present time. Simply reconnecting to your heel bones goes a long way to recovering your equilibrium.

Poise and presence necessitate being in the present moment. Only then can you pivot physically or intellectually in whichever direction you please. This is the freedom that allows you to behave with grace under pressure.

We all live by our feelings so nervousness and anxiety are unlikely to go away but their impact can be lessened if you cultivate these attitudes. The build-up to performance either on stage or for an audition demands a singular focus, taking you outside of the everyday. It is the other emotionally based distractions, habitual stress-related reactions or genuine unpreparedness that introduce a different element of unhelpful stress.

With the help of the technique you can still make a choice to take the panic out of fear. F.M. called this "Staying in touch with your reason". If you didn't learn it before, ask your teacher to teach you the Whispered Ah. This is one of those invaluable exercises that, if you have made friends with it, will propel you into performance freely moving and fully charged.

The Whispered Ah (not be confused with the Silent Ah sometimes taught in voice classes) is an exercise F.M. Alexander taught to his pupils. Its success depends on a genuine feeling of amusement/happiness. Achieving this is helped by realising that the sustained Ah is the basic tone of the word laughter in British received pronunciation. To the one who complained he couldn't think of anything funny, F.M. reportedly said, "Well go home and come back when you can".

Collecting funny thoughts is a lifetime's homework. Enjoy![27]

---

[27] In his book *Born to Sing* (2015, Mornum Time Press) Ron Murdock suggests using a kindly thought, which can also work very well.

Kate's Recipe for a Whispered Ah

Thoughtful preparation is very important for this so don't rush. First of all, abandon any idea of doing a Whispered Ah so that your muscles 'step down' from their habitual readiness to perform. Ask your neck muscles to be free of tension. Smell the flowers, but take no special breath before (or after) each Ah.

Remember something that makes you smile or laugh, funny enough that your eyes brighten and your upper lip can move.

Let the tip of your tongue rest against the top of the bottom teeth. Think of the British RP sustained vowel sound Ah as in 'Laughter', 'Marmite' or a sung 'Amen'. Find your own word as a personal reminder

Keep a happy thought in mind. Open your mouth freely like a fish. Whisper the Ah so that it can be heard.

Close the mouth and allow the air to come in through the nose (warmed and filtered) before repeating several times.

Listen and appreciate how the quality of your thinking and intention affects the sound you make.

Moved into your own Rhythm

Sometimes you may not know why you are moved by an experience or a piece of music or poem or a performance. It is important to be able to stay with this feeling, unexplained as it may be, and to let it travel with you in your store of impressions and inspirations.

All matter vibrates at different tempos. You have a vibratory response to particular combinations of this invisible factor that also equates to the rhythm of your life force or energy (akin to the vital rising sap of a maple tree). It is possible that you have become immersed in a rhythm, dictated by circumstances, that does not match your own deep personal rhythm. At some point you probably adopted this other rhythm in order to survive! A little like birds forced to sing louder in built-up areas in order to be heard above the traffic noise.[28]

Whether or not you were born and brought up to it or transposed from the country or a small town, living in it you dance to the beat of the city. It is often a borrowed tempo and may not adequately resource your potentially expansive self.

Connecting to your own personal rhythm makes it easier to choose how to reveal the inner pulse of any character you play. Take the opportunity to revisit your innate inner timing when you can. Often this requires a stepping aside, a slight slowing down, saying no to further action. (Maybe you have rehearsed this with starbursts of stopping during waking hours.)

Now, whether in a comfortable café, a meditation space, a

---

[28] 'Birdsongs Keep Pace with City Life: Changes in Song Over Time in an Urban Songbird Affects Communication' (2012):
https://www.sciencedirect.com/science/article/pii/S0003347212000541

walk amongst greenery, whatever you need, let the recollections of these experiences begin to move you back into your own rhythm. You can make sense of them from that place. They are a key to your development as an artist.

Sometimes conscious understanding can take years; at others, it can arrive in an inspiration of realisation. I still don't know what combination of factors – whether the cadence of the words or the rhythm – caused me at age 14 to be so exhilarated by my first encounter, during an English lesson, with the poems of T.S. Eliot. I couldn't understand them at all, I only knew that there was something very important in them for me. Certainly, my own love of poetry was born in that classroom. [29]

Several years ago I was helping friends look for a dog's lost ball in a field and found myself standing still, unexpectedly moved by the sight of a tree and had a profound sense of the transmutation and dispersal of energy upwards being facilitated by trees. I wrote a poem about it on a now lost scrap of paper.

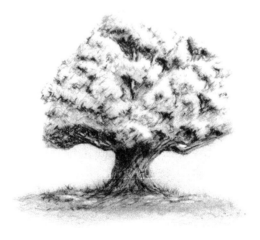

29 T.S. Eliot asserted that we don't necessarily have to understand the content of a poem (that would come later) but the musicality of the thing: "the music of poetry is not something which exists apart from its meaning" [*The Music of Poetry*, 1942].

In 1984 (after a personal crisis) I had become tired and disillusioned with theatre, and felt disconnected from my own rhythm and creativity. I visited an exhibition, a retrospective of the works of the painter Marc Chagall. In the Royal Academy galleries I turned a corner and entered a room devoted to one huge canvas, 'A wheatfield on a summer's afternoon', a backdrop for the ballet 'Aleko' painted for a New York company on tour in Mexico.

In one fell swoop I remembered (though not in words) why I had become an actor in the first place. My faith in theatre and myself was restored, I was close to tears. I was so grateful to Chagall.

It is very evident to me that he was an artist who created from his heart. That is what I responded to and needed to experience and understand in that moment. More recently, visiting Tudeley parish church in Kent and seeing all of Chagall's 12 stained glass windows (the last installed in the year of his death, during that exhibition) was a joyful confirmation of this.

His granddaughter, Bella Meyer recounts[30] that, "The first time I was really in love, he came to me with the biggest smile and said, 'I know now you understand my paintings.'" A floral designer, she later added, "He taught me that each piece I do [needs] to 'speak from the heart'."

He was able to sustain his commitment to an open heart, which remained unobstructed at the core of his life-rhythm and his art, till the end of his days.

They will probably stay in your mind but it's a good idea to record, in words or images, the instances of being moved, however fleeting, for your own notebook of inspirations. These recollections remind you to remain linked to the pulse of your inner life, the ultimate source of your creativity.

---

[30] Masha Leon (April 29, 2011) 'The Story of Chagall, as Told by His Granddaughters': https://forward.com/news/israel/137374/floral-designer-bella-meyer-reminisces-about-her-g/

Whatever moves or touches you will inform the consciousness of your heart and consequently your mind.

The new discipline of neurocardiology[31] has provided the insight that the heart and nervous system do not simply follow the brain's activity and direction.

As significantly as the mind in the spine and Upledger's take on intelligent protein molecules, neurological impulses generated by the heart's nervous system are sent to the brain and 'cascade' up into the brain's higher centres where they can influence perception, decision-making and other thinking processes. "Its elaborate circuitry enables it to act independently of the cranial brain to learn, remember, feel and sense."

The heart appears to be sending meaningful messages to the brain that it not only understands but obeys! Not to be confused with 'emotional intelligence' (more likely to be used as a tool for getting on in organisations and interpersonally) a connection or response from the heart is unstudied, spontaneous and can have a profound effect.

With the heart established as a participant in decision-making, take the opportunity to explore your own heart feelings/ connections while you walk in the park (or on a ramble in the country). Effective intuition in gardening and herbalism is a direct result of repetitive interaction with plants. This is not an intellectual activity. In *The Secret Teachings of Plants*, Stephen H. Buhner devotes a chapter to 'Feeling from the heart' and suggests that the feelings that arise in contemplation of a plant are in fact the healing act rather than the effect of its medicinal properties. Later he also admits that some plants are 'as boring as sociologists' which is his reassuringly humorous way of saying that we don't all have the same feelings for the same things.

---

[31] See 'The Intelligent Heart' (September 22, 2009):
http://alchemyandenergy.blogspot.co.uk/2009/09/every-day-is-peace-day.html

Growing nature is the one continuing live witness to human history. If you are going to play a character in an eighteenth-century play, find a 300+ year old tree. Sit under the tree (phone switched off) and let yourself daydream a little or, if you feel like it, touch the tree and note your physical responses and feelings. Does it engender any particular atmosphere? Seek out a plant that might have been used for cooking or medicinal purposes and imagine yourself into that era and what your dependence on, or use for, that herb might have entailed. These experiences indirectly feed your feeling for the individual you are to play.

A sundial is a reminder of how nature and time have always shared rhythm. Any perception of time passing attunes to nature's enduring clock. Unsurprisingly this significantly influenced social norms until only a few hundred years ago. Sunrise and sunset may have ceased to be as significant for us in an age of artificial light but the behaviour of everyone was affected by the gradations of light and dark, from before dawn to after dusk. The phases of the moon casting inky blackness or causing Oberon to declare to Titania, "Ill met by moonlight" on a full moon night, would have been used in the planning of journeys and outings both secretive and public.

If you are lucky enough to find yourself in a city, town or village observing 'Earth hour' or to be somewhere where street lighting and shop front illuminations are eschewed you may get a better idea of the extent of night darkness during the era of the Restoration and of course in Shakespeare's day.

Experiencing real darkness for yourself makes more sense of the mistaken identities in the bedroom scenario as portrayed in the trick played on Angelo in 'Measure for Measure' set in Vienna contemporaneously with when it was written in 1603-4. It is helpful to know that in 1660 no European city had street lighting but by 1700 it had been reliably established in most major cities in Europe. This radically changed the living habits of city dwellers, so that the evening meal "shifted several hours later" and sleep patterns formerly 'segmented' became more uniform.[32]

But don't forget to look upwards, in city or country. Despite the encroachment of light pollution in most parts of the world at night with a consequent loss of star constellation sightings, in the daytime you will usually see a clear sky very similar (ignoring vapour trails) to that visible in the era your play was written or set. We all feel the difference between a heavy day and a light one. So did our ancestors, the playwrights and the actors in cities and countryside. They also did as you can, lie on your back and enjoy on a clear day the playfulness of the sky's movements.

It is only from a relaxed state that your imagination and thought processes engage meaningfully. Combining your Alexander lying down with a view of the clouds is a fine activity!

As with my exhilarating encounter with Chagall, when I heard Wilfrid Murray playing Chopin at a concert in London in 2011 the only way that I could describe its effect was that my heart felt stretched. There was an expansion. I was moved. The late Bob Moore, the internationally known Irish healer describes this perfectly as a feeling that has growth. Love, joy, understanding and acceptance all have this inherent movement, while on the other hand emotions of fear, anger, jealousy and self-pity will stagnate or contract and will keep, like habits, repeating themselves. Sadness by the way does not inevitably contract unless it is quickly blocked by fear or anger and becomes depressive.[33] A little like the difference between reaction and response, this formula (contraction vs growth or expansion) is a very useful

---

[32] For a wonderful book, which is my source for much of this subject of 'One man's search for natural darkness in an age of artificial light' see Paul Bogard (2013) *The End of Night*, Fourth Estate.

[33] Anna & Alexander Mauthner (2013) *Conversations with Bob Moore*, Moore Healing Association.

way to differentiate between what is most helpful to your heart and imagination, creativity and life and what is not.

Olga Averino the Russian opera singer writes wistfully of a time (not so long ago): "Before airplanes became the main means of transport, [when] there was time between engagements, and even if it was spent on travel, there was a sense of rest and relaxation. The number of engagements was much smaller and there was no feeling of meeting 'the deadline'. Performing was a happy event."

This pace was much more conducive to the life and wellbeing of the performer, in her case as a singer. "Singing is an expression of life", she reminds her reader, "and if you have no time for your life, how can you sing? Quality always needs time, not only in music but also in life itself."[34]

Quoted in support of the worldwide 'Slow movement' I also like Lily Tomlin's solution "For fast acting relief, try slowing down". Encompassing most areas of living, the movement is concerned with recapturing connectedness and alleviating the stress of constant fast, forward motion in over-scheduled lives.

If you are holding down various jobs to make ends meet, rehearsing all the hours given and staying up late to learn your lines, you may wonder how this or much of this chapter could be applicable to you. The Alexander technique is not just about living up to ideals or trying to slow you down but about making the best of what is available. When F.M. asked his trainee students on his 1930s' teacher training course to look out for his "best pupil" in the waiting room they were disappointed to see a rather bent up little old lady sitting in the corner. He wanted them to realise that it wasn't attaining a particular appearance but how you choose to respond to any stimulus in the moment that is important. It is likely that she did the best she could within her given situation and with

---

[34] Extract from the last chapter of Olga Averino (1989) *Principles and Art of Singing*, Intention.

F.M.'s help could release and expand within her framework.

So if "Quality needs time" can there really be any choice in how you are affected by the little time available to you?

Maybe you often don't have enough sleep? My teacher used to say, "if you wake up in the morning and everything is lousy don't try and brace yourself up. First of all you have to accept how bad things are, then rather than trying to do something to make the situation better you want to prevent things from getting worse. It is only from that place can they gradually improve."

One theatre student was very early every morning cleaning the class studios to help pay her way. She found this tiring, stressful and it affected her studies. During our lessons together we discovered that she could approach the cleaning work differently by *dancing* the washing, dusting and polishing. Being imaginative, persevering and talented she turned this situation right around and flourished.

A level of quality in performance and in a happy life may be easier to find when there is calm and rest. You really can, however, create quality in the time you have available. You have the motivation, excelling at your artistry, planning for performance. Use your conscious thinking attitude and awareness of the needs of your inner rhythm to create as many starbursts of stopping during your working day as possible, so you too can experience that 'there is time enough'.

In the Present Moment

Unconscious habit is automatic and doesn't encourage a 360^0 awareness of being in the present moment. To remain receptive and aware, you, the performer, have to be in the present moment, the here and now, for the audience to stay with you and notice your performance. To be appreciated, you cannot ever afford to lose this perspective even or especially as a 'spear carrier', if you want to develop your craft and your career.

Practise a heightened awareness of what you notice during the day and it will help you register the present here and now. Be wary of remaining 'plugged in' with earphones missing a myriad stories unfolding around you, all fodder for your creative storage facility. Michael Billington, the UK theatre critic, recalls a meeting with Laurence Olivier from which he concluded, "that a microscopic attention to minutiae and a Sherlockian fascination with [other people's] physical detail are part of the complex weaponry that makes a great actor".[35]

I learned about truly being in the present moment from my Alexander teacher Walter Carrington, who took over the Alexander teacher training course in London when F.M. died in 1955. However short the amount of time spent with him, there never appeared to be hurry or rush.

Just Meijer is a talented and successful Dutch actor who, when I first met him at the beginning of his career, had created his 'Theatre of the wind'. It comprised a set, costumes and actor touring on a bicycle with a small trailer

35   www.theguardian.com/stage/2014/jul/11/laurence-olivier-25-years-anniversary-death - Michael Billington's memory of Olivier before a BBC Radio interview, 1982.

creatively unencumbered. Working with what is only essential to express his artistry continues to extend to how he lives his life

Whenever he feels out of sorts he gets rid of possessions, ruthlessly clearing out. This to me equates to a not holding onto the past and not fearing for the future and Just's wish and need to stay in the present moment.

Recently he sent me a description of being in the here and now. This is an extract:

> "In awe and amazement I find myself standing on a vast plain in twilight. The earth is alive and the universe beyond the curvature of the horizons is shimmering. There is no time. There is only me, standing still, looking around. Emptiness as far as the eye can see. It is not threatening, there is no loneliness. There is nothing. And that is all there is. All that space... There is room for anyone and everything, and I understand, that I am facing my next ... here and now moment. I know that I am the sum of all the here and now moments that have passed and realize how futile it is to look back into the past. I am the past. I am the latest, updated version of the story that is me. And not only that .... I am the future too. In the moment I am now facing – where there is nothing – I will take the next step and bring my world to life.
>
> Step by step. So, indeed, there is no past, no future ... nothing like that, on that vast plain all around me."[36]

---

[36] In *The Spell of the Sensuous* (1996, Random House) David Abram relates a similar experience: "I remain standing on this hill under rippled clouds, my skin tingling with sensations. The expansiveness of the present holds my body enthralled. My animal senses are all awake – my ears attuned to a multiplicity of minute sounds, the tiny hairs on my face registering every lull and shift in the breeze. I am embedded in this open moment, my muscles stretching and bending with the grass. This present seems endless, inexhaustible. What, then, has become of the past and the future?"

What I find helpful to prevent myself being pulled into the next moment before I have fully inhabited the present is to physicalise the here and now by connecting to my heel bones. It's likely I was already leaning forwards on my toes. This also works to prevent me from thinking of the next line I have to say, being drawn towards the audience, ('please like me, please understand me'), or being absorbed into another person's pattern of posture or expression.

I don't mind repeating that the heel bones are a performer's best friend and these chunky bones really want to support you and are designed to take your weight. When you are too far forward towards the next moment, your knees and lower back tighten, as does your neck, and your head is thrust backwards (chin up) to stop you overbalancing forward. (Too far back and a similar scenario, the same gripping of the neck and holding of the head). Recover the 40/60 tripod of weight-bearing and your head finds its balancing point more easily and the legs don't have to work hard to hold you up. It's amazing how the decision to think in this way can begin to change your mindset and develop access to your own personal creative space, physically grounded in the present moment.

Injury or illness may appear to be strange bedfellows with 'the present moment'. Pain or discomfort, however, if not extreme, focus the mind on what is essential. When you have to work while unwell there is little energy to spare to dwell on either the past or the future. The effects of aging may bring about the same focus while in activity.

Rather than waiting until you are incapacitated, practise honing your attention. Notice yourself in activity, and experience the difference between distraction and conscious awareness. One dissipates your energy, the other energises you.

The following is similar to the exercise of continuing to sing one melody while someone beside you tries to 'put you off' by singing in a different key. It is a game based on an 'eavesdropping' exercise where two people simultaneously converse on different subjects with a third person who engages in these two conversations without losing either thread. Each person takes a turn to be the third – a terrific way for the third participant to demonstrate ability to focus and respond in the moment.[37]

On your own you can read out loud some inconsequential text (i.e. an undramatic weather report), at the same time as listening to a short, recorded story. Take your time to breathe appropriately, speak at a reasonable pace and volume and continue to maintain your balance on your feet and the poise of your head.

Perhaps start with short passages so tensions don't creep in unnoticed. Rigidity does not have to be the inevitable result of increased focus.

Afterwards summarise the story you heard. This is fun to play with and will increase your ability to stay alert to what is important around you while remaining in the present moment. You might gradually increase the interest of the text you are reading to see how much you improve your 'eavesdropping' skills!

---

[37] Most theatre exercises have multiple authors. This is adapted from a 'Kiss' company warm up.

The Spaces In Between

F.M. Alexander located the space between the stimulus for action and actual engagement and saw its great value in giving the individual the tiny slip of time to ensure they can freely choose how to respond.

Others have also noted this space. Philippe Petit talks about what he has named 'Paranoia trees'. "By imposing a delay, by offering a pause", they allow him to see ahead, to anticipate, to avoid something, perhaps underfoot.[38]

Entrenched habit is something the Dalai Lama believes follows a person when in the Buddhist tradition they reincarnate. If I can be forgiven for putting this into a very different context, *The Tibetan Book of Living and Dying*[39] perfectly describes the space available when habit is prevented from jumping ahead of what could be the as-yet-unformed creative impulse:

> There exists always a space or gap before any emotion begins to arise. That pregnant moment before the energy of the emotion has a chance to arise is a moment of pure, pristine awareness, instead of embracing the 'emptiness' of that gap, in which we could find the bliss of being free from, and unburdened by, any idea, reference, or concept, we grasp at the dubious security of the familiar... driven by our deep habitual tendencies.

Actors whose improvisations appear 'samey' are more likely to be reacting rather than responding to the situation.

---

[38] Philippe Petit (2014) *Creativity*, Penguin.

[39] Sogyal Rinpoche (2002) *The Tibetan Book of Living and Dying*, Rider.

Although the dictionary definition doesn't differentiate very much between them I find it helpful practically to think of them as having quite different 'textures'. Unless conscious awareness and choice are implemented, the quick 'reaction' is based on the familiar and dominated by extra muscle tension, especially a stiffening of the neck. The almost-as-quick 'response', on the other hand, teases out the space in between the stimulus and the action, freeing the neck muscles at the same time as allowing something possibly new to arise from that 'empty space'.

If you are walking and behind you someone suddenly shouts your name, the surprised reaction is to sharply twist the head round while at the same time tensing the neck and contracting your breath. Instead try inhibiting any reaction so that you can stop and, in the pause, think of freeing your neck and choose to turn the head with the eyes leading the way. This takes a split second longer but gives you the added possibility of continuing the turn, which the head has begun, to face your friend. Remember to look at your shoulder before you look behind and the naturally occurring spiralling movement will be very easy. When in performance you will be either graceful or haughty depending on the expression on your face but definitely worth watching. Turn your head this way while reversing a car and you will access more mobility and are less likely to hurt your neck. As mentioned in a 'A Generous Voice', for various reasons, there currently appears to be a great deal of 'no neck' in everyday life, where there is little separation between the head and the neck in movement. This tendency to unduly fix the head/neck will not do for any characterisation set in a period where poise and elegance were highly valued. Before the Industrial Revolution survival in artisan and agricultural occupations may have also depended on this freedom and mobility in movement. The actor must be equipped to make the choice to portray what is needed. If you are habitually tightening and stiffening your neck in everyday life, you are unlikely to be able to make the creative choice beyond habit for the characterisation and will find it uncomfortable to sustain if asked to by a director.

So it is useful to familiarise yourself often with the gentle head turn, (in practising, always go towards one side and also then the other, so as not to habitually favour one side over another).

Of course, musical harmony doesn't exist without spaces in between the individual notes. The inhabiting of a rest in a music score is understood with exquisite sensibility in what has been referred to as 'The Wrist Respirate', where Chopin advises the piano player to delicately raise the wrist at the point in a piece of piano music where, if sung, a singer might take a breath.[40]

This awareness of breath is a singular attribute of a space in between. The violinist Tom Eisner is convinced that faulty breathing is responsible for strained nerves in the orchestra pit.

> The most beautiful music ever written breathes, so surely there is something wrong when musicians themselves forget to breathe.[41]

There is a lovely quote from *The English Patient* which I have used many times in workshops to illustrate how much, with the use of computing and texting, we may have forgotten

---

[40] True to his principle of imitating great singers in one's playing, Chopin drew from the instrument the secret of how to express breathing. At every point where a singer would take a breath, the accomplished pianist [...] should take care to raise the wrist so as to let it fall again on the singing note with the greatest suppleness imaginable. To attain this souplesse is the most difficult task I know. But once you succeed in doing it, then you laugh with joy at the beautiful sound, and Chopin exclaims "C'est cela, parfait! Merci!" As quoted in Jean-Jacques Eigeldinger, 1986, *Chopin: Pianist and Teacher.*

[41] Tom Eisner writing in *The Guardian* newspaper, 20 August 2014: www.theguardian.com/commentisfree/2014/aug/20/stage-fright-addiction-classical-music-alcohol

some essentials about space and time when approaching the written word.

The Canadian nurse is reading from Rudyard Kipling's' *Kim* to the English patient:

> Read him slowly, dear girl, you must read Kipling slowly. Watch carefully where the commas fall so you can discover the natural pauses. He is a writer who used pen and ink. He looked up from the page a lot, I believe, stared through his window and listened to birds as most writers who are alone do. Some do not know the names of birds, though he did. Your eye is too quick and North American. What an appalling barnacled old first paragraph it is otherwise.[42]

Practising reading out loud prose or poetry written before the advent of typewriters in general use (about 1874) gives you a better opportunity to find space for unhurried breath as there is a chance that, just like with Kipling or Chopin, the rhythm of the author's own breathing is extant amongst the phrases and punctuation.

A doorway can be a very practical illustration of a space in between. Unthinkingly, we all pass through doorways, framed spaces, perhaps dozens of times a day. It is possible, however, that at the very back of your mind they symbolise portals into the unknown and if the unknown holds any residual anxiety for you, you will react accordingly, albeit with a very slight tightening of muscle. If you can stop and think and choose before you habitually fall through the door (probably with head retracted), each one offers a choice as to how to pass from one place to the other. They become a space in between other spaces. In order to occupy this place in the moment between exit and entrance, play with the following exercise with or without a door in front of you. In it you take a step back to take a step forward.

---

[42] Michael Ondaatje (1992) *The English Patient,* McClelland & Stewart

Begin with one foot behind you (a small step). Check your neck is free and head poised and that you are breathing! Think of going upwards. Don't fall down into your hip in moving. Your front foot can now be 'empty', you could lift it off the ground without losing balance as it is the back foot that now carries your weight. Now, perhaps counter-intuitively, step off with the weighted back foot to move forward. This way you really take your back with you.

If it helps, after playing with the above movement, try thinking of pressing down on the big toe of this same back foot, as though ringing a push button bell on the floor, to flip your foot outwards. This will also activate your knee to release forward. Although as you do this the 'front foot' becomes the 'back one' taking your weight, don't hurry to transfer weight. The 'new' foot now taking front position can make choices as to how to land. Then you continue walking as you choose. Every now and then (in the exercise) stop and repeat the instructions.

If this seems complicated, play with swaying backwards and forwards – again swopping which foot takes your weight until you feel confident balancing mostly on one foot. Then use the simple first version, without slowing down, of quite easily taking a step back to take a step forward. Practise, of course, before trying it in performance!

As always you can ask a teacher to help you with this.

The stimulus of the doorway, instead of beckoning you to pass unthinkingly through, is now a new reminder to consider taking a step back in order to move forward into the new space. Be sure, however, in opening a door that you do not cling onto and even lean on the door handle. As far as possible separate that activity from continuing to walk through the door.

Having prevented an outdated habitual reaction to whatever doorways unknowingly represent, you can sweep through the double doors of a palace, shuffle into the cell door that locks behind you, stride onto a football pitch...

whatever your character's situation suggests. Practise your new relationship with these magical doorways as you enter rooms, offices, railway carriages, supermarkets, exit into gardens, onto pavements... anywhere, so that entering on cue from the 'business' off-stage will become hugely informed and imaginatively appropriate.

Learning with Your Teacher

At the centenary celebration in 2004 of F.M. Alexander's arrival in the UK we were told by Walter Carrington that when F.M. was your teacher you knew you had a friend.

In other words, someone who was on your side. The same method is taught by every teacher in varying ways depending on training, life experience and personality but certainly encouraging a learner is the favoured approach. Alex Bingley told me:

> I never leave a lesson feeling got at, or that I've failed and it reminds me of a quote I read in which Walter Carrington said something along the lines of "Good God people can't go around upsetting other people. They're upset enough as it is" and he's so right.

Philippe Petit has a similar approach when teaching beginners high-wire walking. One of his students relates, "He acknowledges when you do something well and he is encouraging when you don't do something well." A participant is asked to ring on a bell whenever Philippe particularly approves of their movements. No one is left to feel stupid or a failure.[43] Fear reflexes are so easily activated and when we are afraid we can learn very little.

I, and most Alexander teachers, trained for four (or, in my college, five) days a week having the hands-on equivalent of up to four individual Alexander lessons a day. The training is very practical and focuses on the trainees' own use of

---

43 Emily B. Hager (12 August 2010) 'Learning to Walk in the Slippers of a High-Wire Artist', New York Times City Room blogs: https://cityroom.blogs.nytimes.com/2010/08/12/learning-to-walk-in-the-slippers-of-a-high-wire-artist/

themselves in thought and activity. In a painstaking process the unnecessary habits of tension embedded in layers of muscle and also prevalent in mental attitudes are filtered out. Over this length of time the technique can bring about profound mental or emotional shifts in the individual as well as physical changes including in glove and shoe size, a small increase in height and sometimes bra size!

Although an initial course of lessons may not be concentrated and long enough to effect such significant changes, the conscious recovery of your own natural poise can be transformative. Your teacher will have experienced many of the ups and downs of the process you can go through while having your lessons. I should emphasise that these dips and peaks are not expected to be a stormy process but changes that can be felt either in quite a creeping-up-on-you, subtle way or not recognised at all until suddenly, at one point, things fall into place. Despite some advertising misnomers and 'alternative' contexts, your teacher is not a therapist nor medically qualified (unless they also happen to be doctor) and does not treat you or attempt to cure you of

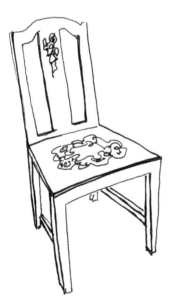

any ills. You are a pupil 'in class' being taught a self-help method.

In the first half of a course of lessons you may feel or have already felt a slight awkwardness or discombobulation as you begin to think about the technique in everyday life, a frustration at not being able to emulate the experience that you have in a lesson and also the tendency to hold onto the 'right way' of sitting down onto a chair, standing up or positioning the head even when you have learned that there is no 'right way'. This particular phase can be mistaken for 'the way of the

Alexander technique' where the holding on produces a stiffening and what I would call an 'Alexanderoid' aspect. A theatre director once confided in me that he didn't like the Alexander technique for what I came to realise was this very reason. He saw some actors moving stiffly on stage constrained by a misperception of trying to achieve an elusive (and eventually fixed) 'right' position of the head. If someone stops taking lessons at an early point they can literally become stuck with this misunderstanding of the technique. As it won't bring them any further towards their goals they will be left with a disappointing experience and perhaps a life time's aversion to the technique.

Change is never comfortable and for some people it takes quite a lot of courage to step away from the familiar and to make the sort of choices offered in their Alexander lessons. It is important, however, to realise that your teacher will never try to force change upon you nor in fact any sort of release from muscle tension. The hands-on work of the teacher along with verbal guidance are mere suggestions to your system. If the sought-after release and change are to happen, they will do so in their own time, with your conscious and unconscious permission, without you or your teacher having to push for it.

People train as Alexander teachers for many reasons including having in turn themselves experienced marked health improvement or an augmentation of skills such as musicianship. One of the other things that may have led your teacher to commit to training is the experience of an enhanced sense of themselves and their qualities while taking their first course of lessons.

Sometimes we don't know what the learning of the technique has done for us until we are in a familiar situation, but we respond differently from 'normal'. After my first course of lessons I discovered that the quality of my stage fright was very different. I was excited and nervous but I could no longer call it fear or stress.

Teachers don't stand still in their learning. They are frequently dealing with the unknown, challenging themselves, looking at their life and their pupils with an outlook refreshed by new experiences. As life moves on, change does not necessarily become any easier for anybody.

Each challenging performing role you take on demands that you face an aspect of the unknown or the unfamiliar, in yourself. When you can use the technique to prevent habitual anxiety holding you into old patterns you release a corresponding creative surge. This can be the reward for accepting the unexpected/the unknown/change for both you and your teacher.

Usually you find the right teacher for you.[44] You may be referred to a teacher by someone you know, or find them through a website or recommended on other social media. If for any reason you find yourself not feeling comfortable with your new teacher or encounter a personality clash and decide to stop seeing that person... please don't give up on the technique but try again with a different teacher.

It may also not be the best time in your life, for whatever reason, to be committing yourself to learning the technique. I have had new pupils booking their first course of lessons 10 years after they first encountered the technique at an introductory workshop or talk! As a performer, however, if you haven't already had lessons (or only a scattered few) I urge you not to wait much longer. You want to enjoy the transformative process as soon as possible to aid and abet your creative life. Individual lessons, the best way to learn the technique, will usually last between 30-50 minutes. Depending on location, rent to be paid and other expenses many teachers will offer a sliding scale of fees or 'special offers' but all will be happier to discuss a concessionary rate if you can commit to a series of lessons.

---

[44] See the Society of Teachers of the Alexander Technique website: www.alexandertechnique.co.uk

For a discounted price I currently ask pupils to take their first 15 lessons within a month/5 weeks. The closer together you have your lessons the easier it is to overcome your strong habitual patterns of habit and to facilitate change. F.M. usually taught his pupils every weekday for a fortnight then another and then another (sometimes with breaks in between). A total of 30 lessons. This is still the gold standard number to learn adequately how to apply the technique to everyday life (the basis for all other creative exploratory work with the technique).

Sometimes the total price for this number of lessons is equivalent to a good holiday. Unlike a holiday, however, the benefits can last you your lifetime.

The Man in White Spats

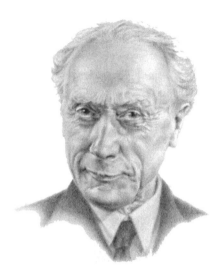

Having assumed, on his arrival in London in 1904, the lifelong role of an English gentleman in his manner of living and dress, F.M. Alexander continued – long after their Edwardian heyday – to wear white spats, not as some thought as an affectation but as a genuine attempt to keep his ankles warm and protected from the draughts in cold English houses. I can't confirm that he and T.S. Eliot ever met although they certainly had mutual friends. Despite the 1939 dedication "To the man in White Spats" in *Old Possum's Book of Practical Cats* it would be fanciful to think that Bustopher Jones (who had "such an impeccable back") – the remarkably fat cat in white spats – could have been based on F.M. but who knows the way a poet's mind works?

Whimsical speculation aside, it is certain that Frederick Matthias Alexander was a performer and as such he understood an actor's energy, that in order to shine brightly you have to 'step up'.

Non-performers do not always understand how, despite illness or tiredness, the actor can metamorphose into an enlivened figure. Adrenaline plays a large part of course. Jerzy Grotowski talked to his actors about the possibility of plugging into the universal accumulator (of energy). The power of Intention is also a strong propellant. Doctor Theatre is renowned for accompanying the actor, feeling poorly, onto the stage.

Tiredness and illness, however, won't be held at bay forever. There are a vast array of methods claiming to conserve energy and support vocal and physical agility, which is why F.M. had to navigate his way through some of the faulty techniques he had learned in order to discover what he needed to continue his acting career successfully.

In 1892 he lost his voice after performances with hoarseness persisting. When rest did not effect the cure his doctor hoped for, F.M. set about discovering what he was doing that was causing his problem. To attempt this without 'expert' help was probably a result of the circumstances of his upbringing. His family had lived in an isolated part of Tasmania where the nearest township was 12 miles away by horseback on rough tracks. As a matter of survival, self-sufficiency was essential. Born on 20 January 1869 at Table Cape, he was a sickly child who became a questioning, precocious schoolboy. He was taken under the wing of a local schoolmaster who imbued him with a love of Shakespeare

F.M. had first taken to dramatic reciting at the age of 6 as easily "as the birds sing".[45] Two decades later, so enamoured

---

[45] F.M. overheard speaking about his youth and quoted in Walter Carrington (1946) *A Time to Remember.*

was he of the theatre that on her tour to Melbourne he went twice a day to watch 'the divine Sarah' (Bernhardt) on stage for the duration of her stay. He recalled these performances for the rest of his life.

When he could afford to, having taken lessons in acting from various teachers including James Cathcart, formerly of the London company of the son of the great Shakespearean actor Edmund Keane, he launched himself as a solo performer, to some acclaim. "Mr Alexander possesses a splendid voice, remarkable for its resonance, power and sympathy", reported the *New Zealand Observer* in 1895. By 1899 *The Australasian* affirms that F.M. was "commendable both for what he does and what he avoids doing". Having overcome his own difficulties, and by this time living in Sydney, he was teaching other performers his method. He was friendly with doctors whose TB patients he had also helped, and became known as 'The Breathing Man'. He was urged to go to London, the centre of empire at the time, to share his discoveries. Money was all that held him back.[46]

In 1904, however, having won an audacious £5 'double' bet on a 150-to-1 outsider in the Australian Cup and Newmarket handicap, he sailed to England on his winnings. He wrote the first of his four books during his two-month voyage on the White Star line 'Afric' but, in exasperation with his first attempt at writing about his work, threw the manuscript out of the porthole before arriving in harbour. He established himself in rooms in Victoria, London where his local grocery was the food hall at the then world-famous Army and Navy stores. His love of horses never left him and he would ride his own horse regularly in Hyde Park and later at his country home in Kent. Apart from one eminent ENT consultant, it was not so much the medical profession but the

---

[46] For an excellent biography (a source I use in this chapter) see Michael Bloch (2004) *The Life of Frederick Matthias Alexander*, Little Brown.

actors such as Viola Tree, the eldest daughter of Sir Herbert Beerbohm Tree (the founder of what became the Royal Academy of Dramatic Art), Lily Brayton and Sir Henry Irving who immediately showed their appreciation for F.M. and his skills. He would go round the West End dressing rooms, particularly the Adelphi, giving them a little 'lift' before they went on stage.[47]

In the period that he gave Sir Henry Irving lessons, F.M. recalled that he stood in the prompt box at every performance he gave in his last London season in 1905. For other actors, including Matheson Lang, he often took the same position, letting his presence remind them of what they had learned from his hands, bringing his observations into his ongoing work with them. Irving's son (Harry Brodribb Irving, also an actor) commented: "He had brains in his hands, and it was an amazing fact that you could somehow understand inexpressible things as his sensitive fingers pressed, pulled and suggested."

It wasn't until 1931 that, at the urging of his supporters, he began a training course in London for teachers. He trained and qualified 45 teachers, nine of whom later started their own training courses including Walter Carrington (my teacher) who continued the running of F.M.'s training course on his death in 1955. He always thought his work would die with him so he might be surprised to know that there are well over 4,000 teachers in different countries, scores of teacher-training courses on different continents and that a great many music and theatre colleges and conservatoires employ Alexander teachers, worldwide.[48]

Although he had relinquished the life of a professional

---

[47] To gain a vivid insight into the world of Victorian and Edwardian theatre with which F.M. was so familiar I recommend a visit to the home of the late great Ellen Terry (Irving's acting partner for 20 years), at the National Trust's Smallhythe Place, Kent, England

[48] See the Society of Teachers of the Alexander Technique website: www.alexandertechnique.co.uk

actor, in 1932 and 1934 F.M. hired both the Old Vic Theatre and Sadler's Wells from his friend Lilian Baylis. He produced 'The Merchant of Venice' and 'Hamlet', casting himself in the title roles, the rest of the company comprising his training students. His aim was to show how his technique could prevent stage fright and enable even the untrained actor to have sufficient vocal ease and poise to face an audience. Perhaps he also wanted, at the age of 64, to have a last chance to play those wonderful roles.

The Daily Telegraph theatre critic wrote, "It certainly speaks well for his methods that his pupils were able to bear themselves with such confidence and to speak so clearly that their manifest lack of stage technique was discounted". The writer also remarked of F.M.'s performance, "There was balance, rhythm and intelligence in every line he spoke."

In his lifetime, F.M. wrote four books – all still in print.[49] Having recovered from a stroke in 1949, he continued teaching until a few days before his death when after a visit to the races he caught a cold and fell ill, dying peacefully at home in London aged 86 on 10 October 1955. Although a kind man, F.M. did not suffer fools gladly and would readily admit to a short temper. According to John Skinner, his secretary and an Alexander teacher, he possessed "a terrific force of personality, even ferocity". After a suitably satisfactory lesson, it is recounted by Walter Carrington that a pupil had walked out onto the pavement cheerfully and thoughtlessly pulling his head back and down onto his neck when he heard a window open and a book hit him on the side of the head. Turning round he saw F.M. glaring at him from the window. "What did you do that for?" he asked. "You know perfectly well why I did it!" was the cross reply. This when F.M. was in his eighties.

---

[49] *Man's Supreme Inheritance* (1910), *Constructive Conscious Control of the Individual* (1923), *The Use of the Self* (1932), *The Universal Constant in Living* (1942).

Stop, Wait, Create

F.M. Alexander once commented to his niece Marjorie Barlow that he could never 'not bother' about living by his technique: "I dare not", he declared.[50] Without it, of course, his performing career would have faded away very quickly. Once experienced and absorbed, the very practical and self-supporting aspect of the technique soon becomes a necessary life ingredient for the actor.

The following recommendations to stop and wait while giving Alexander thinking directions help to embed the technique in everyday life. The ground is then prepared for the unexpected, the creative choice to be made.

Five things

As it is everyday life that informs performance, my rather prosaic advice to you is this. After your Alexander lesson, pick five ordinary things you do every day such as: picking up your hairbrush, putting on the kettle, squeezing toothpaste onto your toothbrush, tying up shoe laces, putting a key in the lock.

Every time you go to engage in one of these actions stop and think and apply Alexander principles using Inhibition and Direction to then make a Choice to do (or not to do) the action. You can also think of this as 'giving consent'.

It will feel a little self-conscious at first but soon it will become easier, especially with the memory of your teacher's hands to reinforce the experience.

You may decide after all that you don't want a cup of tea or that actually you won't bother brushing your teeth! If you

---

50 Marjorie Barlow, ed. (2005) *More Talk of Alexander*, Mouritz

can remember to stop at all (and often you won't in the beginning so strong is the habitual pattern), what you may notice is that before you even made the decision you were already in 'the mode': your head had moved into a fixed awkward sideways movement to receive the hairbrush, as your thumb was about to hit the electric kettle switch your head had retracted...

As your experience of the technique expands, increase your repertoire of five things to cover lots of areas of life. As changes in any muscle behaviour in the body gradually affect others in the chain you won't have to examine every single movement you make to elicit significant changes.

Preventing these patterns develops a keen and essential awareness of your head-neck-back relationship whenever you need it.

It takes time to achieve this but preventing these patterns in the everyday is the key to raising your performance from acceptable to potentially mesmerising.

The conscious mind can organise many thoughts very quickly and seemingly simultaneously... like varying levels of perception. One thing at a time all at once – a little like a speeded-up version of those old-fashioned station indicator boards that clatter downwards to change the train information. When performing on stage all in an instant you can notice the audience member rustling a chocolate wrapper, see scenery wobbling, realise a cue has been missed, be sincerely in your role, feel the perspiration on your face and, when needed, you can choose to release into an action with Alexander awareness.

Alexander awareness or thinking (giving directions), is not a blunt instrument. You do not have to concentrate so hard to the detriment of anything else. On the contrary, the technique aims to encourage noticing what is happening around you at the same time as being aware of what is going on with yourself: you in your environment, wherever and whenever you are in the present moment. Although particularly useful when there is an on-stage emergency (forgetting lines, scenery not shifting), the Alexander technique is concerned with your preparation for performance. Having had experience of the hands-on work of an Alexander teacher and echoing the repertoire of 5 things in everyday life, here are some exercises to enhance your approach to working on stage or set, radio booth or lecture hall, using Alexander principles.

Five More Things

Bow and arrow

Take up your imaginary short bow and arrow, being careful not to contract and pull down as you swivel your torso and pull the bow taut. Weight on both feet, one slightly behind. As the arrow shoots forward release your knees and take more weight on the back foot, let your hand aiming the arrow move forward. At the same time with a free neck and balanced head, breathe out or sing an Ah sound.

Faith Oakley, one of the world's best student archers, has mastered the art of firing arrows from her teeth. She puts the arrow on the string for a couple of seconds, inhales and then exhales. She pulls back and aims and then lets go with her mouth. You could also have this helpful description in mind.[51]

Taxi

Ensure you free your neck and allow the head to find its poise. When you open your mouth, do not push out your chin to project. Stamp your foot at the same time as loudly proclaiming the Tax of 'Taxi'. The power of your connection with your heel bone grounds your voice to let it soar with the 'i' (ee) being the follow through sound. If you have the opportunity to hail a taxi on the street, try it out. You won't need to stamp your foot but remember your heel bone connection before you call out, and do not lean forward.

---

[51] Reported in Kentucky Eastsidernews.com January 2018. See a video of her at www.youtube.com/watch?v=lj2gCBJDg-4

Sandwich

Remember the torso is like the bread in a sandwich and the spine is the filling. You would like both pieces of bread to be similar length. Not one long at the expense of shortening the other. It's easy to think of the back of the torso only as being 'the spine' and to forget to allow a commensurate release upwards in the front at the same time. Release downwards any holding of the lower back (lumbar) curve. This is more a thought than an action, gentle and imperceptible, a request, not a tucking in of the bottom. Place your fingertips on top of your hip bones (not holding on to your shoulders or elbows, let them fall) and as you allow the breath in, notice the release upwards from your fingertips and then, as you exhale, make sure that the lengthening doesn't disappear. These upward and downward releases are linked and simultaneous reminding you of your three-dimensionality.

If feeling pulled down and as an emergency measure, find a table or surface at hip level, place the finger tips on it (with due attention as above), breathe with release upwards in the front and allow a corresponding downward release into the lower back and a sinking into the heel bones (while allowing the head to recover its balance)

Star

Rather than pulling yourself about with a non-thinking stretch, try this. There is a lovely cross body diagonal pathway all the way along your back and the back of your arms between your fingertips and your opposite foot and heel bone. Look ahead with your eyes and your customary head poise.

Let your feet be close together. Without collapsing down into your hip, step your left foot to the side and extend the opposite arm above shoulder level, palms facing forward, taking care not to scrunch the shoulder. Now move the right foot away from the left and extend the left arm, again above the shoulders with palm facing out. Think of the connection from fingertips to opposite heel bone, check that you are breathing and 'twinkle' with hands fluttering like the star you have made. Then turning your arm, only from the elbow (not engaging the shoulders), face your palms downwards to the floor and let your arms float gently down to your sides.

Spiralling

With much talk of going up and lengthening, don't forget that there are no straight lines in nature and that your muscles are spiralling away happily as you move. Face forward with your head poised. Begin walking on the spot with left leg lifting at the same time as your right arm extends forward, continuing with the opposite right leg, left arm, etc. You will feel like a marching tin soldier. Gradually exaggerate the pattern and start moving forward. Forgetting the military analogy, really let your torso twist from side to side but do not pull down into your hips to do so. Now think of yourself more as a fashion model showing off the outfit as three-dimensionally as possible. Keep breathing, think of going up and remember to smile. After a while, to complete the spiralling effect, you could let your eyes lead your head to glance each time at the shoulder which comes forward with the arm. Don't worry if you get into a bit of a muddle at first. Don't force it but come back to it when you feel like it. This is definitely not a formula for walking but an exercise in awareness to play with. The experience can be in the background of your walking and can inform your thinking especially if you suddenly find yourself needing to address any stiffening in movement.

Before the Curtain opens

Alex Bingley observes how easy it is for actors to go through pre-performance warm-up exercises mechanically, in a hurried way, "without truly preparing their voices for the world of the play". Yet he knows that "simple voice exercises achieve resonance, strength and authority when they involve the actor's imagination, heart and gut" – sometimes with unexpected results.

If you find yourself parroting voice exercises without much thought, it might be useful to ponder if there is anything preventing you from a full involvement. This level of commitment of course requires an independent mind, not prepared to downsize into a level of 'norm' that may be around you.

Could, for instance, the smaller expectations of fellow players in some way be limiting your expression? Alternatively, might you still be in thrall to an electronic device recently used and about to be checked again. Are you using the warm up as a displacement activity for nervousness or as a rabbit's foot talisman kind of ritual? Are you anxious that you might sap your energy and tire before a demanding performance?

These mindsets are all deterrents to full participation in the present moment. Remember that energy expended with freedom of thought and action generates aliveness and there doesn't have to be a separation between the quality of your energy in stage or daily life. You can inhabit the present moment from head to toe with whatever unforced vitality is available for your preparation.

LIFE, the preparation for performance

However much you pay attention and keep adding more '5 things' to your repertoire, there are many situations where it is difficult to remember to approach a task or movement with Alexander thinking in mind. Here are a few practical reminders as to how to best use the technique in your life and before the curtain opens.

Lifting

When you go to pick up something from the floor, pay attention to how you are using yourself. Moving props and picking up heavy boxes can all be part of the early (and sometimes later) life of an actor. You need to pay just as much attention to the use of your self when moving the scenery as you do when you are preparing to perform.

You have learned to stop, direct, give permission for the action and then continue to let the head lead in the movement. The neck muscles release and the spine lengthens itself. It is important to remember to stop before the head is 'automatically' retracted. Practise with bags of light shopping. Let them hook in your hand and swing your arm. You can only do this freely if you are engaging extensor muscles that run from the outside of your hand and arm into your back rather than flexor muscles that grip the biceps and tighten your armpit. As far as possible you want to let objects balance in your hand in this way (rather than clenching your fist and tightening your arms to carry them), then you avoid any unnecessary interference with the free movement of the ribs.

Allowing the hips and knees to release as you bend is not a new idea but remember to let the knees go forward and away from each other over the toes. Do not decide at a certain moment that you have released everything far enough and you are in the 'right position' to pick up a bag from the floor. Remember there is no right position. Just like a golfer who 'follows through' with his swing, you want to follow through with this movement, going further than you think you need, to avoid a fixing of joints and a loss of all available flexibility.

If you find, after all, that you have tightened everything up in the effort then be glad you noticed the difference. Use the technique as 'first aid' to stop, check your tensions, let holding fall away, give your directions, recover your equilibrium and start to breathe again.

Learning lines

How you are when you learn your lines is how you will remember them. If you screw up your eyes, tighten your leg in a jigging motion or any other habitual expression of tension, traces of this effortful memorising will colour your learning. Instead incorporate some Alexander thinking into the procedure to increase your absorption and lessen anxiety and repetitive tensing. Practising whispered Ahs from time to time and doing some lying down will also help. Keep an awareness of who you are addressing and the type of space you will be performing in so your eye muscles become used to looking out and your vocalisation is not inappropriately conversational.

Your character crosses their legs

Crossing the legs often tightens the lower back and causes you to pull downwards in front. You will have a habitual and 'comfortable' side you like to cross a leg over. Deliberately choose the unfamiliar side which requires more awareness of what you are doing with yourself.

Arms crossed

Choose to cross your arms the opposite way from usual (this can seem tricky!) and again you will be less likely to go downwards into the chest area and consequently into the hips.

Sitting

In order to use the voice fully, an opera singer when sitting (or lying) has to find the most advantageous position to sing. It is the same for the actor speaking. However naturalistic the play and whatever the status or physicality of the character, you need to seek support from your sitting bones on the chair and avoid shortening the optimum length of the spine.

Practice with various chairs and armchairs at home. Cushions and furniture may be available to use in rehearsal or even incorporated into set design with supportive padding to facilitate unobtrusive uprightness.

Leaning

When your role demands that you lean against something like a wall, you don't have to pull down into collapse, you can find the way to lengthen and release into the pose.

Furniture and Props

When your hand touches the furniture on stage it is very easy to find yourself leaning or holding firm to it. This can easily 'pull you down' towards it. If you choose to place a hand on a table or a chair, use it as somewhere to come 'up' from, to lighten away from, use the connection like a balancing pole. This also applies to carrying a cane or walking stick however reliant on it your character is deemed to appear.

Steps

Your dressing room may be quite far from the stage and involve using stairs. There is a tendency to misuse the knees as brakes while coming down a hill or steps. At home or in a quiet place having decided first of all not 'to do', given your Alexander directions and then your consent to the action, practise with your hand on the banister/rail. Imagine yourself as Charlie Chaplin's 'tramp' in big baggy trousers. Without forcing, let the knees release forward and away from each other over your toes as you let your legs walk you downstairs.

Going up the stairs, again use your Alexander Inhibition and Direction thinking, and with a hand lightly on the rail keep the weight on your back leg for as long as possible without leaning forward when you move up. Spring your back foot and knee forward by pressing on the big toe. This helps to avoid a pulling forward and down and a scrabble to the top of the stairs.

Paper

Despite technological improvements and developments, I don't expect paper scripts to be universally replaced by touch screens. Scribbling in margins, highlighting cues, lines and cuts, and accenting speech breaks all necessarily personalise the performer's script.

Just as with a forward hand and arm gesture it is, however, important to note your imperceptible reaction to holding a script or even a single piece of paper in your hand while sight reading or in rehearsal. Even as you are picking it up from the table or inside your bag become aware of not being drawn towards it with consequential chin jutting and neck muscle tightening. Use your ankles to release away from the strong stimulus.

Audition reminder

You may be in a waiting room with several other auditioning actors. It's too crowded to do a vocal warm up. You won't disturb anyone, however, by making a whispered Ah to warm up your throat, enliven your eyes, facial expression and access your full breath. Notice the doorway to the audition room/stage and accustom yourself to both the thought of it and how you are going to pass through this doorway. If you are sitting, make sure, when you are called, to find your sitting bones before you stand. Don't hurry. An extra few seconds of thought will support your free breathing and movement and help you be your best. Similarly if you are self-taping and it is not your favourite audition method, ensure you practise some whispered Ahs for that very reason and avert any habitual tightening while interfacing with the technology.

Computer

Google glasses and under-skin implants notwithstanding, screen reading is likely to be here to stay. If a tablet or e-reader was to replace paper in the rehearsal room, the 'paper' advice is just as valid and transferrable. If you have spent several hours unthinkingly at a computer and later put your hands on the keys of a piano, you are likely to bring your own unconscious keyboard mode to your playing… so you need to stay aware!

It is also a great temptation to collapse on the sofa with your laptop/tablet while your feet are curled up under you but really it's not worth it for the neck strain later and certainly unhelpful on the day of performance. Introducing the unexpected, like a bunch of sweet-smelling flowers near your computer, can keep you breathing freely and more aware of yourself in the natural rather than virtual world. Stones from the beach and shells to touch can also help to keep you 'earthed'. Before switching on your computer or laptop, notice that you may have already gone into 'computer mode'. Stop and decide not to put your hands on the keys. When seated at a table find your sitting bones and let both feet rest on the floor. Ensure that both arms are parallel or slightly sloping downwards. Check you are not already jamming your teeth together, holding your breath or narrowing your eyes. The next time you become aware of yourself you may be in the old staring, twisted and pulled down position; don't despair, be delighted that you noticed and simply stop and begin again.

Texting and gaming

Both can involve much use of the thumbs. If speed is compromising your shoulders into a held position, and causing you to hold your breath, stop then slow down before you start again. As a reminder to breathe freely, consider singing or humming when concentrating for intense bursts of time.

Although phones/tablets now use much smaller screens than the computer or laptop, all the habits connected with a computer will easily be present. It is hard to resist the omnipresence of a screen phone especially if it is your main means of electronic communication. Check how you hold the phone to your ear (rather than bringing your ear to the phone as though it is on an old fashioned fixed line). Even if using ear phones when holding it in your hand does your body contract towards it?

Charmingly called a 'Handy' in Germany, make sure its very convenience doesn't fool you into ignoring any potential disturbance it can cause you.

Sewing

You may need to do your own mending or even making of costume or perhaps you repair or create your own clothes at home. When sewing by hand, bring the level of the material as close to you as is comfortable to use a needle and thread. Rather than crouching over the piece of work, when it is placed on a cushion on your lap or on a table you are less likely to suffer neck and back ache.

Writing and reading

A writing (and a reading) slope (referred to as the Victorian laptop) may seem hopelessly out of date. It is not so long ago however that all school children (me included!) sat at sloping desks. I am writing this book (both in long hand and typing) seated at an old sloping school desk because it makes it easier for me to write without tensing or slouching forward and down as I write. More people are standing to work and well known authors write standing or alternate between sitting and standing. In the public area of the British Library in London there were standing desks with supporting standing 'chair backs'. If they are still there I recommend having a go if you are ever passing.

When I read, I prefer to tilt the book or e-reader upwards. As with sewing, I am adapting the environment to suit me rather than the other way round.

When reading for pleasure or for work, experiment to find the easiest way to maintain comfort and poise. Without having to equip yourself with specialised furniture, sit or stand at a table, place a book behind the book or reader you are perusing and hey presto it will be on a slope. As with sewing, when it is on your lap, you can bring what you are reading towards you on a cushion rather than leaning over it.

'Inner Ballast' Coda

F.M. Alexander's 'Inhibition' is not designed to keep you in the wings for an immoderate amount of time nor to paralyse your impulse. There must come a time of action. You have given yourself a terrific springboard of 'groundedness', upward direction and freedom to venture forth onto the stage, or set, in response to your cue.

The Czech playwright, prisoner of conscience and former President, Vaclav Havel, did not hesitate to display this courage in art and life, "Vision is not enough", he famously declared, "it must be combined with venture. It is not enough to stare up the step; we must step up the stairs".

The technique is there to support your acting and performance – not to dominate it. It has been part of your approach and preparation not only for the role but also for life... the two being indisputably linked.

As an actor, you are capable of an awareness of all that is going on around you and with yourself. The technique fine-tunes your consciousness to cope better with distractions or 'disasters' and to focus on what is most important in the moment. A most interesting spectacle for an audience is the actor-still, 'composed', poised and free. It is in that instant that the attention you paid to yourself both in daily life and in rehearsal brings a quality of authenticity or even charisma to your presence on stage and screen. In the preparatory hour, or half hour, before the curtains open, or recording begins, you do all sorts of ordinary everyday things like lift a cup to drink, clean your teeth, brush hair, put on shoes and costume.

When you focus on 'before' and apply Alexander principles to your thinking and approach, these activities will no longer be a source of unnoticed tension for you.

You may even start to cultivate a response to the idea of doing these actions that instead frees the neck and releases tension in that area. Your normal pre-performance nervousness becomes less heightened.

Much of the Alexander 'Before' work prepares you for your creative decisions and actions. It supports your energy and calms nerves. Gradually you may notice that the Alexander technique has some special meaning in your life.

Remember, if you are lucky enough to have been born healthy, all the freedom of thought and action is something you and your muscles will have already experienced when you were very young. Accurate and reliable muscle memory is being evoked when you employ Alexander thinking. This then becomes the reliable foundation on which to develop and support your talent and artistry, whatever performance methods you learn. You can use it as the energiser to propel you forwards, beyond any apprehension, into the creative space.

On BBC Radio 4's 'Desert Island Discs' in 1996 the philosopher Professor George Steiner spoke of the amount of poetry he had learned by heart. This, for him, would be 'inner ballast' to support him in his solitude on the island.

I have appropriated this wonderful phrase as for me it describes rather accurately what the Alexander technique can provide, enough inner ballast for you to face the unexpected without being thrown off balance, a practical surety that encourages you to follow unerringly the swerves of the path ahead.

On hearing what this book was called, a colleague joked, "Well we'll know the title of your next book!" *After* may be mine to write in the future but, in the meantime, it is yours to happen. I wish you fulfilment and joy of it.

~~~~~~~ ~

With grateful thanks to the actor and explorer F.M. Alexander and my many teachers and colleagues whose words, styles and knowledge I have absorbed and unwittingly made my own.

All inaccuracies are, however, mine alone.

Kate Kelly
Lac-Etchemin in Québec and London, 2018

About the Author

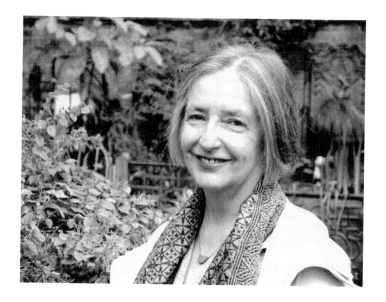

Born and brought up in Northern Ireland, Kate Kelly graduated as an Alexander technique teacher from the Constructive Teaching Centre in 1988 and continued as a teacher trainer there for 17 years. She maintains a private teaching practice in Central London where she lives with her Québecois husband. They both sing in the local community choir she co-founded in 2013.

After Queens University Belfast she performed in Dublin at the Focus and Project, toured with Isosceles theatre and was part of the Lyric Players company in Belfast before attending the Webber Douglas Acting Academy in London. She went on to work as an actor, and later an Alexander teacher, in the Netherlands, France and other countries in Europe as well as the UK.

Along with teaching in drama schools for several decades,

Kate was a partner in Hart Training (now Midderighvox) for 11 years, with Johannes Theron and Ivan Midderigh, bringing theatre-based team and presentation coaching to business and organisations worldwide.

She is a certified practitioner of the Alfred A. Tomatis listening method and most recently has trained as a Soul Midwife with Felicity Warner giving Tender Loving Care workshops on accompanying the dying with awareness.

Kate enjoys organising and giving poetry readings in performance and is passionate about books and libraries and bookshops. She actively supports the movement to keep all local libraries open.

Also from Triarchy Press

Body and Performance edited by Sandra Reeve
12 contemporary approaches to the human body that are being used by performers or in the context of performance training.

Attending to Movement: Somatic Perspectives on Living in this World edited by Sarah Whatley, Natalie Garrett Brown, Kirsty Alexander
Somatic practitioners, dance artists and scholars from many fields cross discipline borders to explore what embodied thinking and action can offer to philosophical and socio-cultural inquiry.

A Sardine Street Box of Tricks by Crab Man and Signpost
A guide for anyone making, or learning to make, walk-performances.

Ways to Wander edited by Claire Hind and Clare Qualmann
54 intriguing ideas for different ways to take a walk - for enthusiasts, practitioners, students and academics.

Nine Ways of Seeing a Body by Sandra Reeve
Nine different approaches to the human body as seen in movement, performance and psychotherapy.

The Wisdom of Not-Knowing edited by Bob Chisholm and Jeff Harrison
Essays on psychotherapy, Buddhism and life experience.

www.triarchypress.net

An inspirational, informative and invaluable book, that brilliantly explains the application of the Alexander technique to theatre artists or anyone keen to improve their physical and mental wellbeing.

Jim Ennis, Co-Artistic Director,
Earthfall Dance

Before the Curtain Opens offers useful insight about how to access consciousness and flow of the body to enhance an actor's performance onstage and off.

Natalie West, Ensemble member,
A Red Orchid Theatre, Chicago

Before the Curtain Opens takes the reader on a lifetime journey with the author Kate Kelly, from her early years as an actor, to the discovery of, and later teacher of the Alexander Technique. The book illustrates Kate's informed understanding of working with actors over many decades and the role the Alexander Technique plays in actor training. Drawing on her observations and teaching many performing artists, Kate's book should be read by fledgling (and seasoned) actors as they embark upon a career that will place great demands on their well-being on and off stage. A general audience can also read the book, as "we are all performers in the act of living." Although not a "how to" book, Kate amply illustrates the many ways the actor can apply the Alexander Technique to help release unwanted physical habits, free the voice and increase stamina.

Dr. Philip Johnston teaches for the Dance and Theatre
departments at the University of Illinois Urbana-
Champaign. His cross-disciplinary courses include the
Alexander Technique for actors and dancers.